How to Survive Trauma

I was heartened by Dr. Colodzin's work. His thought on the communication process, anger and healing encouraged me to feel a sense of belonging and hope. This book needs to be read by all who have suffered trauma in their lives as well as by those who work with and love us.

Christina Crawford, author of *Mommy Dearest*
former Commissioner, Los Angeles County Child Protective Services;
Founder, Survivor's Network.

Dr. Colodzin has organized a very easy-to-read survival kit for those with post-traumatic stress and their loved ones—techniques for personal recovery that validate the reader's dignity.

Cindee Grace, N.D.
Director, Multiple Personality/Dignity (an educational organization)

Beautiful, excellent, and very useful.

Patricia Norris, Ph.D.
Clinical Director, Voluntary Controls Program, Menninger Clinic

This is an extremely valuable and important aspect of treatment for veterans who need a continuum of various traditional and alternative approaches because of the complexity and severity of their problems. I am pleased to support and endorse this offering of "alternative" healing and treatment approaches that go beyond the traditional office-based therapist-to-client "talking therapies."

Raymond M. Scurfield, D.S.W.
Post-Traumatic Stress Treatment Program Director,
Veterans Administration

While reading your book I was struck by the idea that most Russian people I know, including myself, have experienced at least some post-traumatic symptoms. The problem of social adaptation is the problem of our society on the whole, and your book will contribute greatly to our understanding of the problem.

Irena Savelyeva
Russian translator of *How to Survive Trauma*

This books helps us do our work.

Valeri Mikhailovski, M.D.
Director, Center School of Rehabilitation
(Afghanistan war veteran treatment center, Moscow)

HOW TO SURVIVE TRAUMA

A PROGRAM FOR

War Veterans & Survivors of Rape, Assault, Abuse or Environmental Disasters

---

Benjamin Colodzin. Ph.D.

P·U·L·S·E

Station Hill Press

A P.U.L.S.E. Book, published by Station Hill Press, Barrytown, New York, 12507.
Cover design by Susan Quasha.

Distributed by The Talman Company, 131 Spring Street, New York, New York 10012.

This work is a revised and expanded edition of *Trauma and Survival: A Self-Help Learning Guide*, published by Ghost Rocks Press, Laramie, Wyoming. Copyright 1989 by Olympia Institute.

Note: For information about the programs and activities of Olympia Institute and their availability in your area, contact:

> Dr. Benjamin Colodzin
> Olympia Institute
> P.O. Box 750
> Bolinas, California 94924

Library of Congress Cataloging-in-Publication Data

Colodzin, Benjamin. 1954-
    How to survive trauma : a program for war veterans and survivors of rape, assault, abuse, or environmental disasters / Benjamin Colodzin.
        p. cm.
    ISBN 0-88268-119-2: $9.95
    1. Post-traumatic stress disorder.   I. Title.
    RC552, P67C655 1992
616.85'21—dc20   92-35269
                                                                              CIP

Manufactured in the United States of America.

Contents

Acknowledgements

First and foremost, I would like to acknowledge that nothing in this text is original. I have simply organized a great deal of information that was passed on by others. So many people helped in the development of this book that it would require another book to properly thank them all. Gratitude goes especially to my family, to those concerned friends who were willing to discuss this subject, and to all the trauma survivors and family members who shared their truths. Thanks to all of you for the trust and love.

Introduction

Experiencing strong reactions to strong and terrible events doesn't mean you are crazy. In order to survive demanding circumstances, any human being will develop exceptional ways of coping.

This book is dedicated to the journeys of those whose lives have been affected by encounters with the violent side of human nature. I'm writing this book based on my experiences as a therapist in Olympia, Washington, where I worked from 1984 to 1987 with approximately 90 Vietnam veterans and their families. I became aware during this time that many male trauma survivors were in relationships with women who also acknowledged the presence of overwhelming events in their lives. I learned that paying attention to the relevant experiences of my clients often included attending to events as diverse as military combat, childhood violence, sexual abuse, natural disasters, and toxic chemical and biological exposures. In many large institutions, appropriate therapeutic strategies acknowledging the relations between prior overwhelming events and current health were not available. For many trauma survivors and their loved ones, a real measure of peace is not yet possible.

Working with that group, I found that those trauma survivors who practiced the ways of thinking and applied the self-help methods suggested in this book achieved a greater understanding of what had happened in their lives. This understanding enhanced their ability to make meaningful choices. Along with that gain, there was frequently a reduction in the generally recognized symptoms of post-traumatic stress disorder: the intervals of anger and anxiety, sleep disturbance, emotional numbing, substance use, depression, dissociative "flashback" episodes, need to isolate, and others.

This book is written for people who have survived truly overwhelming events and have not yet healed. It is designed to aid the search for ways to live that are more balanced, that enable day-today life to be experienced more comfortably and with a greater sense of control.

For better or worse, gaining such control requires greater self-understanding, along with an increased awareness of one's mental, physical, and emotional reactions under various conditions. This process takes time. It takes a degree of concentration on the details of one's life that is sometimes difficult, sometimes painful.

I have addressed this book primarily to the reader who is a survivor of trauma. If you are such a reader, it is an invitation to embark on a journey to learn more about yourself by hearing the testimony of others and learning better ways to pay attention to what's going on inside you. In practice, this may mean anything from noticing when your jaws clamp tight, to realizing what is happening when you "fly off the handle" after someone you care for criticizes you. I make the basic assumption that the more you learn about how "you" really tick, the more comfortable you will be in your life and the greater the peace you will find in it. **Most of the ideas and exercises presented in this book will be effective only if you are willing to admit there are still important things to be learned.** If you believe that you know all that you need to know about your life, you will be unable to learn from the messages you are constantly receiving from your body, your feelings, and your thoughts. Most of us indulge in a very popular method of not paying attention to ourselves: it is called "denial."

Denial is what happens when, for any number of reasons, we choose to fool ourselves about the information we are receiving. Most simply, it means we edit the available evidence so that it fits into the picture that we are comfortable looking at. When we do this, we wind up ignoring most everything that doesn't fit into our picture.

Let's examine this idea by way of some examples:

Much evidence has accumulated over the twentieth century that would indicate that societies must shift towards sustainable economic development policies or the global environmental degradation now underway as a result of overpopulation and poor choices in the stewardship of resources will make matters far worse. Yet, we ignore much of the evidence that tells us this is so. We do this because to make changes carries many risks and would mean we must alter the picture of the world with which we are comfortable.

Another example: The official U.S. Government position at the Rio environmental summit of June, 1992 denied the seriousness of currently measurable global warming and ozone depletion effects to such an extent that the U.S. voted alone — in opposition to every other conference participant from around the world — against taking immediate and substantial action to cut emissions from damaging chemicals. We are not yet comfortable, it seems, with a picture of the world in which industrial policies have seriously damaged the ability of the earth's biosphere to sustain life, though evidence supporting this is clearly available. Denial is a very powerful tool for resisting change.

Again: Some hundreds of years ago, a popular European myth taught that the earth is flat. While this myth was believed, not much encouragement was given to explorations beyond certain points or boundaries of the known world because this mythic picture denied that there might be profitable consequences to journeying beyond those boundaries. Here again we see how denial can influence choices and allow something that is real and tangible to remain unseen and hidden.

In military history this has been demostrated even more simply: if you don't like the message, kill the messenger. That policy has the effect that no one will be very anxious to reach you with bad news.

For a last example: In a family system, frequently the family member who first points out dysfunctional aspects of family life (e.g., Daddy is hurting the children; Mommy is usually intoxicated) becomes the focus of rage and blame within the family system, "the one who has a problem." Here again we see how energy can become bound up in reinforcing and defending a policy of denial, in avoiding a picture of the world that is true but with which we are not comfortable.

Denial can influence the choices made by nations and individuals. Many trauma survivors have reported that the process of living through their overwhelming events was so intense as to change the way they felt about themselves and their place in the world. The reality of the events imposed certain changes necessary for survival; changes in ways of thinking, feeling, and behaving. Many sexual abuse survivors — upon returning to participation in "normal" activities within their family system — learned that much of what they had experienced did not fit into the picture their family system was comfortable looking at. **Now, if you act on something that most everyone else wants to ignore, then you are likely to make a lot of people uncomfortable.** If you find that paying attention to some of the things you know makes most people uncomfortable most of the time, pretty soon you may learn to deny those parts of yourself, perhaps even to doubt that such knowledge is worth knowing. And when this occurs, you may lose confidence in your ability to teach yourself anything valuable.

If you are feeling an overwhelming emotion while you are caught in a threatening situation, what can you do? One frequent strategy is to learn a style of acting in the world as if those feelings aren't important, are not something to pay attention to. With repetition, it could appear that one had lost the ability to feel at all. We will look at why these responses might happen and what can be done to change them.

All of which is to say that denial, as a way of protecting ourselves from realizations that are painful or otherwise threatening, can sometimes help us survive and at other times can get us in a lot of trouble. In my experience, trauma survivors grow ready to engage the types of inner questioning offered here as they became more willing to explore the possibility that whatever happened before may somehow be connected to what is happening in their life now.

Post-traumatic stress has been called a sane reaction to an insane situation: experiencing strong reactions to strong and ugly events doesn't mean you are crazy. In order to survive, any "normal human being" (whatever that means) when placed in extremely demanding circumstances will develop exceptional ways of mentally coping with the situation. Many of what modern Western psychiatry and psychology describe as the symptoms of Post-traumatic Stress Disorder in trauma survivors are in fact ways of thinking, feeling, and acting that were essential to survival in such extreme situations.

Useful as these "combat mode" styles were for surviving in a war zone (whether the war zone in question might be an Asian jungle or a sexually abusive or alcoholic family), they are generally less useful in creating a peaceful life. In addition, they are misunderstood by and frightening to the majority of those who have not had such life experiences. All of this has contributed to the sort of difficulties we are going to pay attention to. If you accept that post-traumatic stress reactions have become part of your behavior, it means you are willing to say to yourself: "There are reactions that sometimes go on inside of me — in my feelings, in my thoughts, my ways of acting — that have something to do with my 'combat reflexes.' **Sometimes I may react to situations happening now in a way that was useful in survival situations, even when what is happening now isn't a question of survival.**"

There you have it in a nutshell. The biggest thing any of us are up against in learning more about ourselves is our own ability to deny the facts. Frequently, we deny those facts that are painful to remember, those that make us feel ignorant or helpless, and those that cause us to see ourselves as basically "not a good person" (whatever that means to us). This book attempts to make it easier for you to honestly pay attention to what you find as you go on this journey to learn more about yourself.

The assumptions I make as a starting point are these:

1. No matter how much you know, there is still plenty about which you are ignorant;
2. No matter how competent you are in some areas of your life, there are aspects of living that you cannot control;
3. No matter how out-of-control you may be in some areas of life, there are aspects of living in which you are competent;
4. You — like all humans — are neither pure saint nor pure sinner, but somehow manage to have streaks of greed, ego, and hate blend with streaks of self-sacrifice, truthfulness, and love to form your character.

If what you've read so far makes sense, then you are in the position to use what is offered here. This book develops a way of thinking and a set of tools designed to assist individuals who have lived through overwhelming and extraordinary experiences to understand what has happened, to search for meaning, and to use the meanings that are found as a basis for making choices leading to greater peace. It's that simple, and that hard. Along the search, you are likely to re-encounter some of the best and some of the worst in your life.

This book intends to provide a helpful method of looking at trauma and change generally. I don't expect — or want — anyone to accept that this material is useful just because I say it is. If these ideas are helpful for you, you will feel them work, in time, and then is the appropriate moment to accept their value. I ask you to keep an open mind in trying out these tools for change. In so doing, you will increase your opportunities to acquire some skills that can help you live with yourself more comfortably — perhaps even with occasional joy.

Remember: you may be starting out quite comfortable with your certainty that the world is flat. Times change, and so can you.

1

Looking at Trauma and Change

It is important to understand that your condition has developed for specific reasons. These reasons can be seen clearly as you become a serious student of the pattern of your life.

People most often choose to go to therapy when their attention is focused on something uncomfortable in their lives. Somewhere inside there is a perception that behavior is not under control, that some part of the self is not working acceptably, that some lack of balance is present. A person may be seeking more peace, more strength, more control, greater balance, more painfree moments, etc. This perception of imbalance is the basic reason people come to therapy — whether their major concern is with marital problems, anger episodes, or anything else. In short, people seek therapy as a way to help change happen.

In particular, many individuals who have lived through overwhelming events report that they first sought therapy when they found their attention focused on uncomfortable imbalances in their lives. This particular pattern of discomfort has been given a medical name, "Post-Traumatic Stress Disorder," or "PTSD" for short. I will be discussing PTSD throughout this book. However, I do not like to use the term Post-Traumatic Stress Disorder since it is not always useful to think of this pattern of functioning as a medical disorder. Therefore, when I am discussing PTSD, I will drop the "D" for disorder and talk about "Post-Traumatic Stress." This change is not meant to imply that Post-Traumatic Stress does not have serious medical consequences: it does. I make this change from the accepted medical terminology because it makes it easier to concentrate on the person who has lived through something overwhelming rather than on symptoms of a disease. Also, when we look at a person who has lived though something overwhelming and we explain what we see in language that only describes a medical disorder, there is a tendency to focus upon what is wrong with that person, and we might miss much of what is quite healthy.

Because human beings are very adaptable, we change in response to what's going on in our lives. **We change in the ways that help us survive in whatever environment we find ourselves.** People who live high in the mountains develop large lungs to soak up enough oxygen from the thinner air. Most of us develop specific defenses inside our bodies to protect us from the types of germs we take in from our food, water, and air every day.

Because trauma survivors by definition have been exposed to an environment highly unusual by modern American mainstream and middle class standards — an environment where the behavior required for survival is very different from what is considered normal or appropriate in the United States — many have developed ways of behaving appropriate to the nonpeaceful environments of their experience. Such behaviors may have been imprinted very deeply and may still continue in the present.

General Patterns of Post-Traumatic Stress

Let's take a look at the signs and symptoms that help you know how to recognize when post-traumatic stress is present. What does it mean when we say a person has "got" Post-Traumatic Stress? First, we mean that this person has lived through something traumatic, namely, something intensely frightening that is not the sort of thing that happens to everyone. **According to the psychiatric definition, a traumatic event is an event "outside usual experience."** Remember that "usual experience" is a culturally relative term; this means that how unusual any particular event is depends in part on what you were experiencing before it happened. One common quality of all traumatic events is that they force a person to place a very focused kind of attention upon what is happening. This intensification of focused attention is a state of consciousness that is unusual compared to the states of consciousness a person normally experiences under nonthreatening conditions. Whether based upon a single overwhelming event or an entire life history of such events, the pattern of action and self-protection that we call post-traumatic stress is connected to real events that have been experienced to be profoundly threatening to the integrity of self.

Living through a traumatic event or series of events is not the whole story about post-traumatic stress, however. It is a necessary part of the picture; it is the overall situation, including what was happening "outside" in the individual's environment, as well as what was happening inside in the person's reaction to his or her experiences, that made the effects of the traumatic events so severe.

Each individual reacts differently; any particular event "outside usual experience" may seriously upset one person and not upset another. An event may also disturb an individual at one time but not at other times.

When we are talking about "post-traumatic stress," we mean that an individual has lived through one or more traumatic events that were psychologically overwhelming, that were so different from previous experience or so intensely painful that the individual had an extremely powerful and uncomfortable reaction to what happened. It is a natural and healthy action of the human mind, in such circumstances, to take steps to ease the discomfort. Therefore, people who feel this type of reaction often make some very basic changes in how they deal with the world in order to cope.

To emphasize how natural and how important these changes are for our mental comfort, let's look back at the psychiatric definitions again. They assume that any event that rightly could be called "traumatic" would be overwhelming to most people; that is, it would be "normal" to have a strong reaction, to be knocked off-balance in some way by what happened. In the case of minor trauma, feelings of anxiety and related symptoms usually fade within hours, days, or weeks. **For major trauma and repeated trauma, strong reactions may continue for years.**

In the case of modern-day combat veterans, it is well known that sounds of helicopters flying overhead or explosive noises can bring on the type of strong reactions that were in fact appropriate in a war zone. In the case of a child abuse survivor with a history of molestation by an alcohol-intoxicated perpetrator, the smell or presence of alcohol can bring on the protective reactions that were in fact appropriate to this type of war zone. Knowing the intense emotions that accompany these reactions, it is easy for us to understand that a person may develop all kinds of ways of thinking, feeling, and acting that help guard against remembering the trauma or the feelings associated with it. Just as people develop specific immune system reactions to defend the body from being overwhelmed by particular kinds of germs, so too do people develop specific reactions to defend the mind against being overwhelmed by particular memories. An individual who experienced the painful loss of loved ones in a traumatic event might find it tougher now to allow loved ones to get close to the heart. A person who judges that he or she acted irresponsibly during a traumatic event might now find it difficult to accept responsibility.

If you have undergone a traumatic experience, the reflexes activated in order to survive it probably didn't seem very unusual while you needed them. This is so, particularly if the traumatic event(s) lasted more than a few moments. But when you returned to an environment where such reflexes were very unusual indeed, in a thousand ways, directly and indirectly, you were told to stop using the reflexes you had depended on to survive. Chances are that no one told you how to stop; few people would know how.

In the best case scenario, individuals return from traumatizing experiences to an environment that feels "safe," where there is time to think, to feel, and to be silent about what had happened, and also to express these things with loved ones or other respectful listeners. In such an environment there is sufficient room for a person to go through their reactions, sort them out, and then to see what has happened in a way that enables moving on.

Many trauma survivors report their experience to be very different from this scenario. There is often no one to talk with about what it all meant, no "safe" place to be found, and in many cases it seems a lot easier to "stuff" feelings — which means to avoid them — than to let them surface where they might get out of control. In such cases, pressures stemming from unusual and confusing experiences may stay locked inside for a long time.

If you are a person who has had insufficient opportunity for such pressures to be released, your mind and body have likely found other ways to cope with their presence. This is what "post-traumatic stress" most basically means. The symptoms of post-traumatic stress — the uncomfortable experiences that constitute the medical disorder — are really deeply ingrained ways of acting that are somehow connected to the unusual experiences that happened before. The following is a list of some of the medical symptoms commonly found in the disorder:

Symptoms of Traumatic Distress

1. **Vigilance and scanning:** Constant checking on what is happening around you (as if something dangerous is about to happen).

2. **Elevated startle response:** Being jumpy when something surprising happens — as in hitting the dirt when a helicopter flies overhead, or whirling around in combat-ready stance when someone touches you from behind unexpectedly (war zone survivors), or diving away from a window when the ground rattles from a passing truck (earthquake survivors), or experiencing a paralyzing or freezing response after a sexual invitation (sexual abuse survivors).

3. **Blunted affect** or **psychic numbing:** A reduction or loss of the ability to feel. This can include an inability or reduced ability to bond with other people, to experience joy, love, creativity, playfulness, and/or spontaneity. A large number of survivors with post-traumatic stress difficulties have stated that it has become much more difficult to feel these feelings since their exposure to "unusual experiences."

4. **Aggressive, controlling behavior:** Acting with violence. Although usually this means physical behavior, it can also refer to mental, emotional, or verbal violence. More simply, it is a high degree of willingness to use force to get your way, even when it is not a survival situation.

5. **Interruption of memory and concentration:** Difficulty concentrating and remembering, at least under some conditions. Concentration may be excellent at certain times and can be severely interrupted by exposure to any experience that causes a stress reaction.

6. **Depression:** In post-traumatic stress reactions, depression can reach the deep, dark "there's no use in anything" rock bottom of the human heart. Exhaustion, negative attitude, and apathy may be part of this type of experiencing.

7. **Generalized anxiety:** Includes tension in the body (such as back cramps, stomach cramps, or headaches), in the mind (anxious, worried thoughts, "paranoid" fears that someone is after you when it isn't so), and the emotions (sustained feelings of fear, low self-confidence, guilt).

8. **Episodes of rage:** Not mild anger; this refers to violent eruptions such as volcanoes can show. Many survivors who have experienced these episodes report that they are more likely to

surface under the influence of drugs, especially alcohol. However, they also occur without drug use, so it would be inaccurate to assume they are "caused" by such use.

9. **Substance abuse:** In an attempt to control the complications produced by all the other post-traumatic stress symptoms, a significant subgroup of trauma survivors, perhaps especially war veterans with post-traumatic stress difficulties, have dosed themselves with marijuana, alcohol, and (to a lesser extent) other controlled substances. It is important to note that there is another substantial group of veterans with post-traumatic stress difficulties who use only prescribed medications, and yet another group that chooses to use no medications at all. To my knowledge there has been no reliable national study to determine the relative size of these three groups; many veterans with post-traumatic stress have been inaccurately stereotyped by the unclear reporting of subtance abuse as the "real" problem in PTS. Clearly a large number of trauma survivors develop serious substance addictions; many others with serious PTS difficulties find coping strategies that do not include self-medication with such substances.

10. **Intrusive recall:** Probably the most important symptom indicating the presence of post-traumatic stress. Intrusive recall refers to old, usually ugly, memories about traumatic events that come up suddenly, unexpectedly, wham! They are frequently painful, often frightening. These recalls can come both when you are awake and when you are asleep.

Waking intrusive recall experiences mostly happen when something in your environment reminds you of "what happened back then" in a traumatic event: a smell, a sight, a sound that is similar to one from that time. Images from "back then" can come rushing into your mind with strong power, and cause a great deal of stress. The major difference between an intrusive recall experience and a normal memory is the strong anxiety reactions that come with the intrusive recall-type memory. These reactions limit the ability to stay focused and alert in the here-and-now.

Intrusive recall experiences when you are asleep are called nightmares. These kinds of dreams generally occur in two types: In the first type, the dreams replay traumatic experiences to which a person has exposed — almost as if one were watching a videotape of what happened then. In the second type, the scenery and/or the characters in the dream may be very different from those in the original experience — but at least some element of the dream (it may be a person, a situation, or a feeling) will be the same or very similar to an element in the traumatic event.

People frequently wake up from these dreams sweating, tense, and exhausted. The medical literature lists "night sweats" as a separate symptom of PTSD because many post-traumatic stress victims wake up drenched in sweat but do not recall any dreams. However, it is likely that this type of sweating generally occurs as a reaction following a nightmare — whether it is remembered consciously or not. Many sleeping partners of survivors who have observed directly these uncomfortable dream states have reported physical movements where the body reenacts its movements during the remembered traumatic event. These types of dreams are, for those who experience them, among the most frightening and least discussed aspects of PTS; we will take a deeper look at what they might mean and what might be done about them in Chapter 7.

11. **Dissociative "Flashback" experiences:** This is a special sub-category of intrusive recall. A dissociative experience is one in which the mind, while recalling the traumatic event, actually takes some particular form of action as if the event were happening now in order to not pay attention to what is really happening now. A dissociative flashback is an experience in which the memory of what happened then (in a traumatic event) is so powerfully emotionally charged that the mind takes specific action such that what is actually happening now fades into the background and is perceived as less real than the memory. In this type of "dissociative state," a person behaves as though they were partially or completely back in the type of situation they faced during the trauma — using a style of acting, thinking, and feeling similar to the style they used back then to help them survive. An individual with a history of traumatic childhood violence, for example, may in such a state defend against the perceived aggression of those who resemble their family of origin; an individual with a history of traumatic military combat may in such a state defend against the perceived aggression of those who look like their war zone enemies.

12. **Insomnia:** Difficulty falling asleep or staying asleep; in the case of those with intrusive recall-type dreams, it is likely that some individuals don't want to go to sleep, fearing to have this sort of dream. In these cases insufficient sleep leading to exhaustion can also be a part of the post-traumatic stress picture. Insomnia may also be caused by high anxiety levels

with inability to relax, as well as by high pain levels due to physical or emotional injury.

13. **Suicidal ideation:** Thinking about suicide, or planning some action that moves one in the direction of ending one's life. When continuing to live is viewed as more frightening or painful than dying, it can begin to look like a reasonable choice to die. When a person reaches this low point where there are no visible good choices available, this is "suicidal ideation." Many trauma survivors have reported reaching this low point, and it is a national tragedy that so many have acted upon it. Among those who have not, there is agreement that with time and seeking, better choices do become visible.

14. **Survivor guilt:** A feeling of guilt at surviving "unusual experiences" where others did not survive; one of the feelings frequently described by those who have experienced "psychic numbing" (difficulty in feeling emotions) following overwhelming events. Many post-traumatic stress victims will go to great lengths to avoid contact with anything that stimulates remembering the events where such tragedies occurred. Where such feelings of guilt are strong, they may also fuel self-defeating behavior, or what one veteran has called "participating in your own mugging."

These are the basic symptoms and the course of development of post-traumatic stress. If that type of stress condition is present in your life, perhaps by now you have recognized one of the above patterns as pertinent to your situation. In that case, you have learned a name for a pattern that you already were familiar with. In learning to understand more about what has happened, you will be taking some important steps along a healing pathway. I have described typical symptoms of post-traumatic stress not because I feel you need to understand complex psychology or because I want to help you focus blame for your present discomfort onto the past, but because it is important to know that your condition has developed for specific reasons. These reasons can be seen more clearly as you become a more serious student of the pattern of your life.

If you have recognized yourself in this pattern we call post-traumatic stress, that is the essential first step. It means you are ready to be more open about accepting some of what is real in your life. This helps you reach a state of mind in which you can ask the next question (you don't have to have any answers yet): "Is there anything I can do about it?"

2

The Myth of Readjustment

True healing is not a matter of meeting someone else's standards, but of making peace with what is true in one's own life.

The pattern of human functioning that has come to be called "post-traumatic stress disorder" really refers to a particular style of holding one's place in the world. Our society and our scientific community have judged that style to be an illness: the medical community does not speak about "post-traumatic stress" but about "post-traumatic stress disorder." What calling it a disorder assumes is that reducing or eliminating the disease symptoms can be expected to generate a cure, and this is reasonably accurate as far as it goes. However, there is a further assumption: it is also anticipated that reducing and eliminating symptoms will bring a person "back to normal." This means returning a person to an orientation where he or she will once again use a style of holding their place in the world that is within the range of the cultural norm. I call this type of assumption the "strategy of readjustment."

Why "Readjusting" Isn't Enough

There is a problem: the "strategy of readjustment" assumes that the mission of the traumatized person is to "readjust"; that is, to rejoin the flock of mainstream America. By "mainstream America" I am referring to the social beliefs shared by most people in middle-of-the-road America. The problem with this readjustment mission for individuals who have had vast and profound exposure "outside usual experience" is that it may be inadequate to the task of leading trauma victims to a state of greater peace and comfort in living. It can predispose a traumatized individual, for example, to believe that one's mission in seeking health is to "readjust"; that is, to become "normal," to "get with the program" and to stop acting, thinking, and feeling in ways that are somehow different.

What such an approach really offers is a symptomatic form of treatment to help an individual adapt to other people's standards of behavior. I am suggesting that this type of adjustment may be insufficient to generate healing. True healing is not a matter of meeting someone else's standards, but of making peace with what is true in one's own life.

Another consequence of the "readjustment" style of thinking about healing is that it makes it easy for trauma victims who have not stopped acting, thinking, or feeling in ways that are outside what our culture considers "normal" to feel like failures. **In moving towards real healing, it is less important to be acting "normally" than to be extremely honest with yourself about what's happening in your life right now.** If what is happening now is strongly influenced by important memories or ways of acting, thinking, or feeling that belong to the past, then it is important to be honest about that too, whether or not it is "normal" by anybody else's standards. As you come to learn how "unusual experiences" have affected your life, you may also come to regard your task in healing as something more personal and more encompassing than simply "readjusting."

One way to illustrate the limits in the "readjustment" way of thinking is to describe a geometrical puzzle called the "9-dot game."

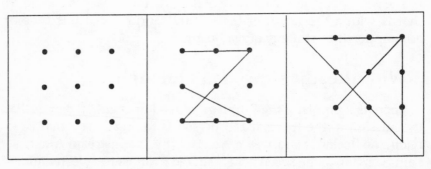

Figure 1   Figure 2   Figure 3

This is a simple puzzle where you are asked to connect nine dots, equally spaced in three rows of three (see figure 1). The task is to connect all nine dots with four straight lines without taking your pen off the paper. If you try to do this, you quickly learn that it is not possible to connect all nine dots with only four lines, as long as you remain within the boundaries of the square outlined by the nine dots (see figure 2). The correct solution (see figure 3) requires that you extend your lines outside the boundaries of the square. Once you learn the solution, it becomes easy to see that only your own mental limitations kept your attention focused on seeking solutions within the boundaries — the solution was always there, available to anyone who was willing to search beyond the seeming limits of the square.

In a similar fashion, "readjustment" approaches to healing tend to apply the values and standards of "usual experience" in seeking solutions to the problems of those exposed to events "outside usual experience." This is somewhat like being unable to draw lines that extend outside the square. Just as the 9-dot puzzle requires a solution that extends beyond the artificial boundary created by our minds, so too may post-traumatic stress difficulties developed by exposure to situations that are "outside usual experience" require healing solutions that extend beyond the artificial concept of "readjustment."

Adapting: An Example

Let me illustrate this point with an example involving one particular symptom associated with post-traumatic stress. This example will focus on the symptom called "vigilance and scanning," which as you may recall refers to a person who is paying extremely close attention to everything that is happening in the immediate environment, a person who is on nearly constant alert for signs of danger. By "normal" American standards this type of behavior is unusual at best, and might perhaps be considered to be the symptom of some mental illness.

Let's examine the situation from a different point of view. For a veteran who has lived for a considerable time in a place where it was frequently not possible to tell the difference between friends and enemies, between places that were safe and places that were not, it would make sense to check the environment with far greater exertion than under less hostile circumstances. There is an old military commercial from the Armed Forces Vietnam radio network played during the war years describing the sounds of a careless American getting in his jeep and starting the engine quickly, followed by a loud explosion and sirens blaring. The commercial ends with this warning: "Check your vehicle for booby traps before you go anywhere."

Now, this type of thinking is outside the usual experience of most of us here in America. We get in our cars, we turn on the ignition, and we don't worry about boobytraps. When a person has lived in a place where survival depended upon drastically different ways of thinking about one's situation in the world and drastically different types of actions, profound changes in one's ways of reacting and behaving can result. This could happen to anyone who found himself in a similarly unusual situation; the sorts of "unusual experiences" that are traumatic are of such a nature that almost anyone would be profoundly influenced by experiencing them.

The warning about boobytraps gives us a reminder of the ways of thinking and styles of acting that were "usual experiences" in Vietnam and other war zones. To return to our symptom called "vigilance and scanning": many individuals who have exhibited vigilant behavior have had the experience of being judged by others as "paranoid," or thinking in a way that is based on unreasonable fear. If we take that judgement in the context of the warning about boobytraps, it becomes easier to see that the boundary line where you distinguish between "reasonable fear" and "unreasonable fear" is tremendously different for individuals with different kinds of experiences.

For a person who has lived his whole life driving his car between his locked garage and the underground parking lot at his office, to habitually check his car for boobytraps would appear an unreasonable fear, because as far as he knows that just doesn't happen to people, really, in the here-and-now of his life. And yet to a person who has had the "unusual experience" of witnessing other humans injured and killed by such lethal devices, it might not appear an unreasonable fear. This person knows it has happened to people, really, in his life. It might in fact seem quite reasonable to this man to exercise greater caution than the other man could understand as reasonable. With this in mind we can begin to appreciate the dangers in reflexively judging the behavior of others, because that which seems an unreasonable fear from one point of view may appear quite reasonable from another.

To say this is not the same as saying that it's just fine for a former soldier, 20 years after his war experience, to be spending a great deal of time thinking boobytraps are about to go off if he's not careful.

We could fairly call this attitude imbalanced and based on an unreasonable fear (unless of course he lives next to a mine field). But what you do about it — once you have made the determination that the amount of vigilance and caution in your life might sometimes be excessive — is very different depending on whether you are using the "readjustment" approach or what I call the healing approach.

Developing a Healing Approach

If you are excessively vigilant and think you need to get "readjusted," you will focus your efforts on stopping your vigilant behavior and trying to be "normal," like the commuter whose experience tells him boobytraps don't really happen. This may not be possible for you to accomplish, since you know something he doesn't know. You may get angry with yourself every time you have a vigilant reaction, judging that you have failed again in your mission to be "normal." If you see yourself as excessively vigilant and adopt the healing attitude towards this imbalance, you will focus your attention upon remembering that at one time you needed to be that vigilant, and that it is easy for you to use that "mode" of behaving again when you are stressed. When you have reminded yourself that this reaction is "normal" for you, you can begin to give yourself permission to become consciously aware when it is happening: "Oh, yeah, there's that uneasy feeling again." **When you know how to identify that a stress reaction is occurring, then you can ask yourself if it is appropriate to the situation:** "Hmmm, there's that feeling in my gut. Is there some real threat here and now, or am I experiencing a stress reaction?"

With this approach, you don't try to be like anybody else. You do the best you can with the ways of knowing that belong to you. You learn to question your automatic reactions and to make them work for you. In this way you can learn to take steps to relax when you react from stress, without losing the ability to retain vigilance and caution when necessary. When you do these things, you are developing a skill that helps you live more comfortably with yourself as you are. **Anything that was learned in your unusual experiences that is still of value to you does not have to be "readjusted" out of your life so that you may heal.**

The best news about post-traumatic stress is that even after many years of confusion, anxiety, depression, etc., it is still possible to find some peace in your life — if you want it enough to work at it. This has been borne out by the experience of many trauma survivors with long-term difficulties. Through learning to understand the effects of one's own "unusual experiences," it becomes possible to see oneself as "normal" even for a person with so much exposure "outside usual experience," and to gain greater peace through acceptance of what has happened.

Healing involves coming to terms with who you are, learning to see change not as an enemy but as an ally. This is the real mission for healing. When you can ask "how can I find meaning in what has happened in my life?", change becomes possible. What happened in the past will not change; it will not become more beautiful or less ugly. But your feelings in the present — about yourself, about what happened in the past, about what it all means — can change. Healing involves opening up new possibilities, new ways to be in the world that bring more peace inside. I have been privileged to watch it in motion many times.

Traumatic Change and Inner-Directed Learning

The biggest problem in using the "readjustment" strategy is that, perhaps unintentionally, it can help people avoid change. When you are using this approach you are not asking yourself questions like "What would it take for me to feel good about being alive in the world today?" — the type of question that might lead to answers about what is blocking such feelings. Instead, you are forced to ask yourself questions like "what would it take for me to be readjusted?" This type of question does not necessarily lead to any insight about how you feel inside or any options for change; rather, it tends to direct your attention to your behavior and how it is not normal.

Consider, for example, such common judgments as "you drink too much," "you get angry too easily," and "you don't let anyone really know you." All of these judgments are based on observations that something is out of balance, yet they all point towards the question "what is wrong with you?" and away from the question of what needs those behaviors might be meeting.

Now, you might choose to change such behaviors as part of your healing process. On the other hand, if what's really bothering you has a great deal to do with old pain and the reflexes you have developed to cope with it, then just changing some behaviors may not bring healing. The "readjustment" strategy says changing unhealthy behaviors is what healing is about, and so it attempts to help people to change them.

The problems come when people developed the unhealthy behaviors (like drinking too much) in the first place to cover up something else that was bothering them. I call this the "Stuff It" reflex — it is a common type of behavioral conditioning among trauma victims. The "Stuff It" reflex pushes your feelings deep down where their emotional impact is felt with less intensity. It is associated with clenching of the body musculature. The problem here is that as you become conditioned to stuffing your negative feelings (anger, hatred, jealousy, rage, suspicion), you lose ability to feel your positive feelings as well (love, kindness, companionship, trust). And it is from your positive feelings — about yourself, others, and life — that you get the motivation and the energy to change what you would like to change about yourself and your situation.

When you are thinking about "readjusting," most of your attention goes to planning how to reach your destination and you don't have to think much about where you have been. This is why the dominant treatment philosophy in American medical centers has not emphasized discussion about traumatic events or the dreams that still recall those experiences. Emphasis has focused instead on a very limited version of the "be here now" approach, where the basic message is to forget the past (reasoning that you can only affect what is happening now).

The inadequacy of the readjustment approach, and the reason I call it a "myth," lies in its ignoring the fact that for many survivors some aspects of what happened in the past are still present in their lives. For them, the emotions are just as though the events are happening now. For such individuals "being here now" has to be expanded to include paying attention to what happened before. **While it is true that it is not particularly useful to dwell excessively on the past, it is also true that our past experiences are our richest sources of knowledge about our own strengths and weaknesses.** Whether we want to remember our past strength or learn from our past weaknesses, we need to have access to what has happened to us before in order to live most fully now.

Unhealed wounds in our memories that block access to our past place limits on who we can be now. It's something like owning a TV tuner with 20 stations available, and on which you can only get reception on 3 channels. The others have too much static. To be whole, we need to learn to be open to receiving information about who we are on all channels. For humans, unlike TV tuners, it is mostly our fear that creates static. As we learn to tune in more and more channels about ourselves, we find we have more and more choices available about how we want to deal with whatever is happening. This means greater freedom and the possibility of more peace inside, even though it may have very little to do with feeling "readjusted."

Natural Change

I like to explain this strategy of healing by referring to a natural phenomenon I have observed at a place where our Olympia Institute occasionally conducts wilderness education events. It is a place high in the California Sierra mountains, on a mountain that has been highly impacted, or traumatized, by human use. There was a silver boom there in 1868, and 3,000 Civil War veterans spent about five years blowing it up with dynamite and extracting silver and gold. The human anger directed at the earth is very evident in this place where 120 years later large areas still resemble a moonscape. Some life has, however, grown back (see photo on page 17).

The interesting thing about this place in terms of this discussion about readjustment vs. healing is that the life forms that have grown back in this devastated ecosystem have been forced to grow in very unusual environmental circumstances. This is pinion juniper wood-land country, and the pinons and junipers that have returned to this scarred and traumatized landscape have not always assumed the shape of "normal" pinions and junipers growing straight and tall. Frequently, they have not been able to do that owing to the special circumstances of their life situation, because the ground has been blasted down to bare rock, and they needed to lay down their roots in unusual "coping patterns" to draw water and survive the high winds of this unprotected area. Many of the trees that have found ways to survive in this area have grown in strange forms: some hugging the ground, others growing with unusual twists and knots in order to meet the demands of their situation. Others growing in shaded areas have tilted their growth in some particular direction where, from their vantage, they can best access sunlight.

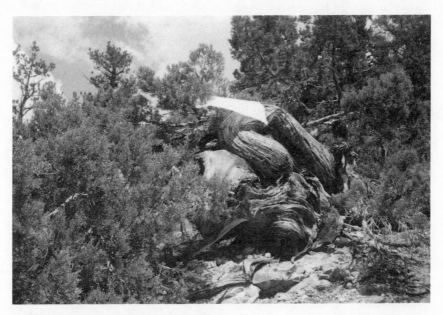

Juniper regrowth following reduction to bedrock by mining, 1868-70, El Descanso Mine, California Mines. (photo: Tsolo)

I have come to believe that there is an important lesson for us humans in the survival story of these trees growing in a traumatized landscape. If these trees had been seeking to "readjust," you see, to be "normal" and straight trees as their mission, then, in many cases, they would not have been able to withstand the pressures in their unusually harsh environment; they would not have been able to successfully reach towards the limited quantity of water or sunlight available from their position. These survivor trees, of course, did not attempt to "readjust"; they were able to send their life energies (roots and branches) out in directions that could support their particular needs for nourishment, whether this resembled anything "normal" or not.

It is my impression that many trauma survivors have likewise reported experiences of having their internal environment "blasted down to the bare rock," creating unusually difficult terrain for life to grow in a nourished way. And so I am suggesting that for individuals with this type of experience it may be highly useful to grow their personal "life-tree" with the lesson in mind provided by the piñons and junipers: **Let in the available nourishment that will support your life, whether this grows you straight ("normal") or in other forms.** Who is to say that a tall straight tree is more beautiful, more healthy, or more normal than these?

Healing comes from honoring what has been learned along the way and applying the knowledge in one's life now. For this reason we will dispense with the notion of "readjustment" and seek instead the choices that may lead towards a life you can respect.

3

Learning to Recognize Fear

Traumatic events are often so frightening that they overwhelm our ability to feel secure about our place in the world. The path to healing includes learning to become aware of and honest about our fear.

In this chapter I am going to ask you to question yourself about how you deal with fear. Fear is real for human beings. It is a part of our lives. For people who have lived through massive trauma, fear may be involved in a big slice of life experience. If we wish to make it a smaller part of our daily lives, we have to learn to know when we are feeling it.

When we were babies, fear was a common part of our lives. It was a feeling that happened naturally when we were surprised by the unexpected or when we were made uncomfortable in some other way and didn't know how to return to a state of comfort. As we grew up and learned about the world, some of the unfamiliar things that had frightened us became familiar and we stopped experiencing discomfort in their presence. We learned to handle other uncomfortable aspects of our lives by behaving in ways that stopped the discomfort or at least minimized it to the greatest extent possible. **Most of us in this country have learned that it is usually not acceptable to handle fear by being honest about it and letting ourselves feel it.**

One of the reasons why so many men who experience long-term PTS have not had opportunities to take an honest look at what was overwhelming in life is because we live in a society where the social code has discouraged that kind of attention to our fears.

When we speak about traumatic events, usually we are speaking about happenings that are not only "outside usual experience" but that are also very frightening, painful, and so intensely threatening that they have overwhelmed our ability to feel secure about our place in the world. If you continue to feel overwhelmed by something traumatic that has happened in your life, the path to healing includes learning to become aware of and honest about what previously frightened you so strongly that it damaged your sense of security.

This may seem like something so simple that it doesn't really need to be learned. Unfortunately, because of our negative attitudes about admitting fear, many of us have become very good at fooling ourselves when we feel it. So we are going to review some of the clues that help us know when it may be present. I will first discuss generally how fear affects human functioning. This may help you to understand how hidden fears can sometimes play an important role in the state of your health.

Fear in the Body

The human nervous system, which includes the brain and all the various networks of nerves, is our central computer system for processing information about what is happening inside and outside the body. This computer also sends commands to the rest of the body, telling all the parts how to act in line with the information it has gathered about current conditions. Without becoming too technical, I want to describe one particular type of command sent through the nervous system. This is a built-in command that gets activated on "automatic pilot" whenever we perceive the conditions around us to be sufficiently threatening.

This command is known as the "fight or flight" reflex. It switches on automatically when certain conditions tells us that threat is nearby — when, that is, we are frightened. When this command is received, a complicated series of electrochemical events takes place within our bodies that affects heart rate, breathing, muscle tension levels, various chemical fluid balances, and a whole lot more. All these reactions taken together comprise the "fight or flight" reflex.

The basic outcome of all this activity is to make a big jolt of energy available to us to face the immediate danger. The more severe the threat, the bigger the "jolt" of energy suddenly made available. **When the "fight or flight" reflex is activated, we do one of two things: we fight that which is threatening us, or we run away.**

Whatever our choice, the "fight or flight" reflex is built into our nervous system in order to alert our body quickly, to help us survive the danger. Throughout human history it has proven a very useful reflex, designed into our nature over a long evolutionary period.

The "fight or flight" reflex, however, cannot distinguish between real and imaginary danger. Every time we believe there is something truly threatening us, even if we are interpreting the situation incorrectly, the "fight of flight" reflex produces a "jolt" of energy. What this means is that the more we feel threatened by what's going on around us, the more our nervous system will maintain a state of high stimulation. This will all be happening unconsciously.

The "fight or flight" reflex becomes sharper the more it functions, and duller when not used. People who feel relatively safe and secure most of the time may not experience more than a moderate "jolt" when they perceive a particular threatening situation, while people who feel threatened a great deal of the time may get a fairly large reaction. When you understand how this reflex operates, you may also begin to understand the connections between traumatic experiences and some of the styles of action associated with those who have lived through them.

According to the accounts of soldiers who shared their stories with me, in wartime Vietnam, threat could be anywhere. There were extended periods where there was no time to safely "stand down," to relax, to act as if your position were secure. In this type of situation, for example, the "fight or flight" command was activated far more frequently than in most situations back home in "usual experience." Combat veterans in the field may have spent most of their waking time with the "fight or flight" command in the "on" position. In this way, a reflex that under usual circumstances is active only rarely sees almost constant activation. A state of extreme alertness and physiological excitation that is unusual in civilian life becomes usual for the combatant.

The nervous systems of people with these types of experiences have, to varying degrees, been trained to transmit the "fight or flight" command very quickly and with minimal stimulation. For example, this is what is actually happening when a veteran who hears a firecracker go off unexpectedly — many years after war experience — jumps quickly for cover with heart pumping and adrenalin flowing. He is using his highly trained reflexes to help him survive. It's just that in this situation, these reflexes are reacting to a perceived threat instead of one that is really present. This is also what

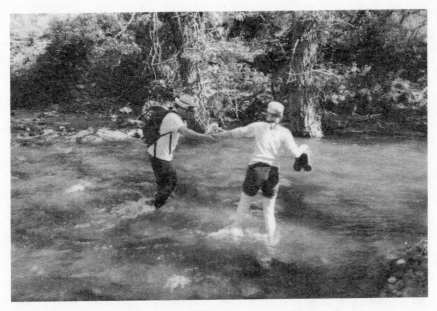

Moving through unstable conditions, California Sierras. (photo: Tsolo)

can happen when an incest survivor who is aggressively bombarded by sexually harassing behavior from a paternal-like figure experiences increased numbness and inability to speak, or an increase in eroticism-related behaviors. She is likewise using coping reflexes that helped in previous survival situations. The connection between PTS and the "fight or flight" command has been clearly demonstrated. Doctors have measured levels of noradrenalin (one of the chemicals released in sending the "fight or flight" command through the body) in the blood of Vietnam veterans with post-traumatic distress that are significantly higher than that in the general population. (To my knowledge, noradrenalin levels in sexual abuse survivors and other trauma survivors has not yet been seriously studied.)

I have been discussing the "fight or flight" reflex in detail in order to explain some of the connections between things that happened "then" and things that may be happening "now." Excessive activation of this reflex can lead to a wide variety of stress-related symptoms including muscle tension, hypertension, depression, irritability, aggressive behavior, "freezing" or paralysis response, sleep disturbance, and anxiety — all of which are associated with PTS. When "fight or flight" has been activated often enough, it becomes possible to send the body this command without knowing you are sending it. Therefore the healing process includes learning to read the signs when your individualized "fight or flight" reflex is flashing general quarters.

Even when the "fight or flight" reflex is over-sensitive, it is still activated only when you are feeling threatened in some way. That is why it is so important to learn to recognize fear: you need to know when you are afraid so you can be aware that at those times you are also participating in sending the "fight or flight" command to yourself. With this awareness you can know when it will be necessary to use fear-reducing methods to tone down the "fight or flight" command and improve your ability to relax and experience peace.

"Clues" from the Body

What are the clues that can tell you when the "fight or flight" reflex is active? First, we'll look at some clues that are likely to show up in the physical body. When the "General Quarters" alarm goes off, heart and breathing rate usually speed up. The muscles become more tense. You may notice increased muscle tension in the jaw or shoulders. If you are holding your jaw clamped tightly shut, this may be a clue to a high tension level. If your shoulders become hunched up tightly and do not drop slightly when you exhale, this may also be a clue to a high tension level. If your hands are clenched into fists, this may be a clue. If your breathing is shallow and you cannot take a deep breath in and out, this may be a clue. Physical symptoms of clenching, tightening, and holding may focus in a particular part or may be distributed widely throughout the body; this is very variable and related to body history. What is common to all such responses is that a "general quarters" alarm will increase the clenching or "holding-on" pattern and increase tension somewhere in the body. This is easy to understand. **When in "primed for action mode," your body doesn't want to unclench fists or jaw, drop the shoulders, or breathe deeply.** These actions would relax the body, and this is not what you are telling your body to do when you're transmitting the "fight or flight" command.

With practice, you can become more aware of these types of reactions in your body and you can learn to become aware of them when they are just beginning. These are the times when it is easiest to change them. It's sort of like having an early warning radar system that can let you know when to scramble your defense forces. Only instead of a system that scans the skies for enemy aircraft, the type of early warning system I suggest you develop scans inside your body and your feelings to let you know when something unusual is happening. Just as a radar warning system is most effective when it gives you the maximum possible time to deal with the incoming threat, so too are we able to reduce the high pressure of a stress reaction when we have more time available to acknowledge that pressure is building.

In the body, then, this early-warning system will be on the lookout for very tight muscles, fast heartbeat and rapid breathing, "jolts" of adrenalin, and the other sensations you experience in your body when you are tensing up. It may take some time to become aware of these sensations, or you may know them very well. If you are not aware of what happens in your body when you become anxious, learning this is a first step. **Go through your body and take inventory, asking yourself what each part feels like when you feel high pressure.** Do you feel your toes are hot, cold, or numb? What about your ankles, calves, thighs, butt, sexual organs, stomach, abdomen, hips, low back, neck, forehead, etc.?

Try taking inventory both when you are feeling calm and when you are feeling pressured. Experience the difference. Use your observation of the difference to help you become familiar with what happens in your body when you are stressed. **The sensations you learn to recognize in your body when it is feeling stressed are among the most important "clues" you can detect about your use of your "fight or flight" command.** You can learn to watch for them, like blips on a radar screen, as a way of detecting when unusual activity is taking place.

"Clues" from the Thinking Mind

We can learn to watch out for thoughts that may be "paranoid," thoughts based on fears that will seem unreasonable once we examine the available evidence. Since the definition of "reasonable" varies between different individuals and within the same individual over time, it can be very difficult to be sure whether an idea with fear in it (fear that something bad is going to happen) is based on reasonable caution or unreasonable fear. There is no firm boundary line; you will have to use your judgement. But with some careful consideration and a little practice, you can sharpen your judgement by learning to test it against reality.

Let me give an example. Suppose you are sitting alone in a big rock formation in the wilderness, fairly relaxed, when suddenly you notice a rattlesnake close by. It has begun to rattle and arches its body as if ready to strike at you. In this situation, the "fight or flight" command would be switched on by most modern people: most of us would perceive the presence of a threat. The snake is poised to strike, danger is definitely nearby, and you need to make some fast decisions. Very few people would judge you to be thinking "paranoid" thoughts for perceiving a threat to your well being. To say the least, it would be reasonable caution to behave in a way that puts some distance between you and the threat, and to do so now.

Suppose it is now several days after your rattlesnake encounter — which you presumably survived — and you are back at your home in a large city. You have never seen a rattlesnake there or heard about anyone who did. Yet every time you walk through the rock garden in your backyard (which looks very similar to the rock formation in the wilderness where you met the snake), general quarters sounds off, and you find yourself filled with adrenalin and scanning for signs of a rattlesnake.

In this situation, the "fight or flight" reflex would not be activated for most people who walked through the rock garden — they would not perceive any threat. You are thinking about an idea with fear in it ("there might be a killer rattlesnake nearby") that is not reasonable, given your knowledge that snakes do not live in the city. You are using the type of caution that was reasonable to use in one kind of experience (wilderness with snake) and applying it to another experience where this amount of caution is less reasonable. This is the type of thought we can accurately call "paranoid." Your body, however, will respond to the "fight or flight" command with the same reflexive "jolt" of energy and tension that it would receive if you were truly in danger.

The result is that you now find yourself with much more energy than you need to deal with what's really going on, and this extra energy will demand to be released. This all started, remember, because you had thought that you were being threatened, here and now, by something (the garden) that wasn't really threatening. When the threat is real, you will, of course, be glad your body is "pumped up" by the "fight or flight" command and ready to respond to the challenge. But when you find, upon taking a hard look, that the threat you initially felt is not really happening now and that your "fight or flight" command has jumped the gun, you will know that you now have to open some safety valve to let out the extra pressure. **Clearly it is very important to learn how to test your fear-thoughts, to learn if the threat they imagine is really there in the here-and-now.**

How do you "take a hard look" and test this type of fear-thought? One really strong test is to ask yourself, as soon as you feel yourself tensing up and sliding into "action mode," a question that can help you get some perspective on how threatening the situation really is. For instance, you might ask yourself, "Is this a life-or-death situation?," or "Is this a question of my survival?"

Let's go back to the example. In the first sequence, when confronting the snake, a real life-and-death situation potentially exists. Improper action could cause great harm or even death. So, when you feel the onset of "action mode" suddenly affecting you and ask yourself if it's a matter of life and death, it takes only a split second to evaluate the evidence, answer "Yes!", and take whatever action is necessary. In the second sequence, when walking past the rock garden and feeling threatened, you may receive an adrenalin "jolt" and a sense of danger that is as intense as the feelings when you faced the snake. But in this situation, when you ask yourself, "Is this a life-or-death situation?" and evaluate the evidence, your thinking mind may see clearly enough to override your fear-thought and enable you to answer "No!" When you can do this, you will begin to reduce the intensity and power of the "fight or flight" command.

If you are a person who has faced threatening circumstances many times, the chances are good that you have trained yourself to react extremely quickly to danger. This may be a source of strength when you face real danger; it can get you in serious trouble when you face an innocent situation that appears dangerous. **By asking yourself the basic question "Is this a life-or-death situation?" you will buy time to analyze situations that are not life-threatening.** This can help you to avoid using your threat-related reflexes when you don't need them. You will also be "reality-testing" your thoughts to see if they are "paranoid"; that is, to decide if they are based on reasonable or unreasonable fear.

For trauma survivors, this type of reality testing may be particularly important because of the possibility of dissociating under high pressure. When something that appears threatening is happening, you may not only see what is going on in the here-and-now, your mind may also remember previous threats that look similar to what is happening now, and you may even perceive the here-and-now as if it were like some threatening experience from the past even when it isn't. This blurring of the ability to distinguish between past and present during threatening circumstances is one reason it is so important to learn to recognize when fear may be affecting your judgement.

Fear and Anger

There is a special relationship between fear and anger. Anger is a reaction to fear. This means that in the places you find anger in your life, something threatening has happened first. Anger is one way to deal with the threat. This does not mean that anger is somehow false or unreal; as you may know only too well, anger is a genuine emotion that we humans sometimes experience with powerful force. When we look at moments when we were particularly angry, we find that before we got to that state something happened that we interpreted as threatening. This applies across the whole spectrum of anger from mild irritation to killing rage. It means that when we are learning to recognize fear in ourselves, the places where anger shows up can provide some powerful clues.

Of course, it's natural and perfectly normal to feel genuine anger when we are truly threatened. But as I have been explaining, sometimes we feel threatened because of unreasonable fears. Threats that are based on unreasonable fears can make us just as angry. **So if you experience a great deal of anger in your life and want to have less, it helps to get better acquainted with the threatening things that cause your anger reactions.** In so doing you will be changing your focus from looking at how someone out there "caused" you anger, to looking at how you are responsible for turning on the "fight or flight" command when something appears threatening. You may never have any control over what anyone "out there" is doing, but you can gain more control over how you react to it. This may be of particular importance for trauma survivors, for it is far better than dealing with events that are outside one's control by ignoring fear, pain, and discomfort.

In military training for combat, it is fairly standard to subject the raw recruit to a prolonged state of exhaustion and helplessness, which gives rise to fear. Once the recruit is trained to obey orders through fear, then information is provided to help rebuild his confidence "teaching him mastery of a variety of skills. He learns certain ways to control his body and his thoughts, to adapt to various environments, to project force, etc. One very important behavior that is taught by example is how to respond when one is afraid. The recruit is shown the model of the "good soldier," who responds to challenge in particular ways. One is expected to imitate this model and suppress one's true response. Incest survivors from dysfunctional family systems are similarly trained not to be honest about their fears, and instead to repress their true selves and behave in accordance with the agenda of others.

Threat, Fear, and Traumatic Stress Reactions

When one is threatened by enemies, it is a very natural reaction to experience fear and to activate the "fight or flight" command to deal with the situation. This sends adrenalin (a hormone associated with the experience of fear) and noradrenalin (a hormone associated with the experience of anger) pumping into the blood, making energy available to fight or to flee. The recruit is taught in such situations to think about winning, about controlling the situation, about overcoming opposition. He (or she) is taught to use the "jolt" of energy that he has experienced to pump up his emotions into an aggressive state from which he can override his feelings of fear and continue to function. This is a time-honored method for helping soldiers prepare to fight in war, and it is very effective for the purpose.

What we are looking at here is one of the consequences that can follow from this combat training wherein you develop a reflex to react with aggressive, controlling force whenever you feel fear. With enough practice, you don't have to think about it, or know that something is making you feel threatened. It just happens. Some fear-producing stimulation, then wham! Immediate aggression: a reflex, without thinking.

This is just the type of anger that many Vietnam veterans with PTS difficulties have described as a source of trouble in their lives: "I don't know where it came from," "It just happened suddenly," "It's as if it happens for no reason." **When anger happens, there are reasons, but they may be hidden.** If you have spent many years living with the type of reflex I have been describing, you may have elevated levels of noradrenalin (the anger-producing hormone) in your blood, and you may have frequent anger episodes that don't make sense to you.

The learned pattern of reacting with fear is different for sexual abuse survivors, although they share a difficulty in consciously recognizing fear-based reactions. Those placed in sexual demand situations under aggression or other fear-based pressures learn a different coping style to support the growth of their "life-tree." In this situation, the individual is usually given little or no opportunity to think about winning, or directly controlling the external situation. She (or he) learns instead to use the "jolt" of energy made available by the situation of the fight or flight alarm to seek escape. Where no physical escape is possible, the survivor is likely to develop an internal escape pathway-into numbness of the physical body with an attendant freezing response, and a state of mind focused elsewhere than the here-and-now. Rather than engaging a pattern of using aggressive, controlling force, individuals with this type of reflex will tend to lose touch with the ability of their essential self to project force. This may result in using a passive-aggressive style of controlling force, which really means mobilizing the defenses against perceived threat using a style that deflects attention from conflict in the here-and-now (rather than resolving conflict). With all the differences between these two very different life experiences, they share a common tendency when under threat: a tendency toward dealing with fear by bringing coping reflexes learned in highly dangerous circumstances to bear on what is happening now, whether danger is or is not truly present.

I have been discussing fear because recognizing fear can help put the brakes on runaway anger, anxiety, body tension, and the tendency to dissociate (to not stay present with what is happening now). Recognizing fear honestly is the first step. Once we can see how our fear has knocked us off-balance, we can begin to consider how to move back towards a more stable position.

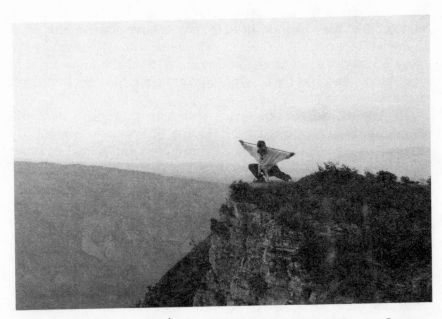

T'ai Chi Master Hussein Magomayev, Hollenbeck-Aoul, Dagistan, Russian Caucasus. (photo: Tsolo)

4

Cultivating Balance

Under ordinary conditions, the discipline of cultivating balance can help you experience a greater measure of peace in your daily life and an increased ability to tolerate stressful events. In the most extreme circumstances, it can be a life-saver.

I have been talking about stress-producing ways that people react to what's going on in their environment. Now I will talk about learning how to shift gears from the experience of high stress and anxiety towards the experience of balance.

What does it mean to be balanced? Some people might say that if you can jump on a pogo stick or do cartwheels, then you have good balance. Others might say that if you keep your cool when the enemy breaks through the perimeter during an attack, then you have good balance. Still others might say that if you can tolerate being stranded in gridlocked rush hour traffic without a stress reaction, then you are balanced. There are many definitions. One thing that virtually everyone who lives in the Earth's gravity field agrees to about balance is that when you lose it, you fall down.

This can be either literally true, as when your body loses its equilibrium, or a figure of speech, as when your emotions or thoughts are running at some extreme that reduces your ability to function. **When I refer to balance, I mean maintaining your equilibrium in a way that allows you to do the things you are trying to get done.** Since human beings have minds, emotions, and bodies all working together, you can lose your physical balance, your emotional balance, or your mental balance. If you physically fall down, for example, it will affect the flow of your thoughts and what you are feeling. If you become very angry, it will affect both the direction of your thoughts and what is happening in your body. So when you lose your balance in any way, it can affect how all the parts of you deal with surrounding events.

Rebalancing

When I speak about the idea of cultivating balance, I mean that it is possible after falling down to get back up and rebalance yourself. In fact this rebalancing is a natural ability that we use every day, though often without being aware of it. Cultivating balance is a useful strategy for anyone who is troubled by their own imbalances, such as strong emotions, absence of emotions, or certain types of thoughts that won't go away. Speaking about cultivating balance does not mean that you need to "get balanced" and then stay there all the time. That is not what human beings normally do. Instead, the strategy of cultivating balance invites you to consider the following idea: **When you fall down, you can get back up again. You can rebalance yourself.**

The tools and methods I will discuss as helpful in cultivating balance are just that: tools, and methods. They are not the only ways to achieve balance. There are many ways, tools, and methods. I will present a few that I have used myself and have seen work for others. They work slowly, over time, and with practice. I present them as useful examples of ways of acting that can help to provide some anchoring in keeping your feet well planted upon the surface below. In presenting this material, I do not wish to convince you that these are the best methods to cultivate balance. I am simply using my own experience to illustrate that the methods that have worked for us in regaining balance can be helpful as we consider this whole notion of overwhelming events and healing.

Learning refined methods of balancing is similar to an experience common to most human beings early in life, namely, learning how to walk. When you first learned about walking, you were very likely quite shaky and fell down easily. You didn't simply decide one day "I will walk now" and get up and jog around the block. Walking took some time and practice: losing your balance and falling down and figuring out what you did wrong. With time, practice, and mistakes, and learning from those mistakes with the determination to know more about walking, eventually your physical sense of balance improved, and the muscles that support the action of walking increased in strength. Walking became much less of an effort, and you acquired the skill needed to maintain that particular aspect of balance.

The balancing strategy presented here works the same way. We will be looking at a method specifically designed for reducing muscular tension in the physical body and at a method for enhancing general balance. If you are experiencing high levels of stress, then for you moving towards relaxation is travelling in the same direction as moving towards balance. This is not always the case. Balance is related to the ability to function within a particular range, where function is most efficient. Not too much energy, not too little. Using the example of learning to walk, too much tension will produce rigid muscles and an inability to walk. Too little energy in the muscles will also prove imbalancing. Balance is not about being as relaxed or as energized as possible; it is about maintaining your composure, maintaining the position necessary to get the job done (whatever the job is at any given moment).

Imagine a modern office building with a ventilation system that regulates the air temperature. Such a system will have some balancing method built into it to keep the temperature within a given range. The system may be regulated so that when the temperature drops below 65 degrees, a thermostat notices the change and a command is sent that blows warm air into the building until the temperature climbs above 65 degrees. The system may also be preset so that when the temperature climbs above 75 degrees, the system also notices this change and sends a different command. This command sends cool air into the building until the temperature has dropped below 75 degrees. This is a mechanical example of the type of system called a "homeostatic" system, namely, a system designed to keep rebalancing itself. **Human beings are partially homeostatic systems. This means that some of our basic characteristics are designed to help us function within a balanced range.**

What you will be looking for in seeking your own balance is the state that you need to return to in order to function efficiently in the tasks you have chosen to perform. In simple terms, when you are balanced you have planted your feet in such a way that what happens in your life cannot knock you off-balance very easily. Concerning post-traumatic stress and this idea of balance, I have found that one frequently reported post-traumatic stress difficulty is a very high level of muscle tension with associated cramps, spasms, headaches, etc. I have many times observed with electro-myographic biofeedback equipment that many trauma survivors hold extremely high levels of tension in particular muscle groups but are not consciously aware that those muscles are tight. In fact, these muscles have in some cases been held tightly for such a long time that the individuals cannot remember what it feels like for those muscles to be relaxed.

In this situation, the feelings associated with very tight muscles are experienced as "normal." On several occasions people who had the experience of learning with biofeedback to relax tight muscles initially reported discomfort because it felt to them so strange and "not normal" to experience those muscles in a state of relaxation. With time and practice, again, change becomes more acceptable. People can learn methods to return their muscles to a balanced range just as the ventilation system in an office building can return air temperature to a balanced range.

Practicing Balance: Push Hands

One of the best ways to learn about balance is by doing rather than talking about it. One highly effective method I have found to de-scribe this general idea of balancing ourselves is through sharing a very old game called Push Hands, which I first learned about from a traditional Taoist teacher. Since then I've learned that many cul-tures have their own variants of this game. The version I will explain requires two people to play.

It is a game with just a very few rules. In the basic starting position, two people stand erect facing each other, about 2 or 3 feet apart, legs spread slightly, toes pointed ahead of the body. You place your arms up in front of you, palms forward and fingers raised (see figure 4), lined up with the other player's hands. Here are the rules. First, you may lean forward on your toes, or backwards on your heels, but you may not move your foot position. If you move your foot position, this is defined as losing your balance (and therefore the game). So the rule is: don't move your feet. The second rule is that you may make contact only with the hands of the other player. If you touch any other part of their body, this is also defined as losing your balance (and the game). You may not hook your hand around the hand of the other player, yank their arm or push it into their body. The only allowable form of contact is between your outstretched hands (with fingers up, palms turned outward toward the other

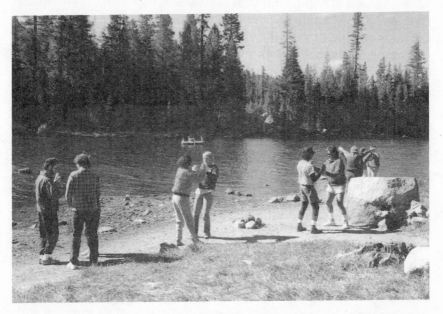

Playing Push Hands, wilderness demonstration for health professionals, California Sierras. (photo: Tsolo)

player) and theirs. You may push as hard as you want to, and you may also move your hands and arms out of the way of the other player.

These are the only rules. Do not play Push Hands if you cannot limit yourself to hand contact: someone could get hurt. If you follow the rules, this is a safe form of contact game that can be played even between people of very different sizes. The interesting thing about this game, and what makes it different from so many games, is that the idea here is not to win by defeating the other person but by maintaining your balance. **The objective is not to make yourself the victor and the other person the loser but simply to avoid losing your balance.** This game can have one winner, two winners, or no winners, depending on who succeeds in maintaining balance. The most favorable outcome is when both players maintain their balance.

When playing Push Hands, then, "winning" is defined as the ability to push outward with your force and to receive the force of the other player without moving your foot position. When you play this game, if you can do these things without moving foot position you are maintaining a certain level of physical balance. **What's interesting about the game is that you can frequently lose your physical balance because of mental or emotional imbalances that come up while you are engaged in playing the game.** For example, suppose in the first round of the game that you pushed forward with great force, expecting to make contact, and the other player simply moved his or her arms out of your way. You came flying forward, off-balance, and the other player laughed hysterically, which made you annoyed.

This annoyance perhaps generated a desire to win, to have the opportunity to laugh at the other player as they just laughed at you. If you get hooked by that type of desire during this game, it will affect how you play. Your desire to win may translate into tight muscles and an imbalanced use of force when you are pushing at the other person. If they notice, they will simply get out of the way again and let you lose your foot position by the power of your own imbalanced use of force. In this way, you can lose your physical balance as a consequence of losing your emotional balance. You can also lose your balance when receiving the force of the other player — if you hold excessive muscle tension in your shoulders, low back, hips, or knees. **This game makes you aware that it is sometimes necessary to bend, to maintain your balance.**

What happens is that you receive firsthand experiences about how your body-tension knocks off your physical balance, and how your thoughts and feelings affect your balance as well. You get firsthand knowledge of how unstable you can become if you lose your calm emotional or mental posture and also where your individual "frozen" or rigid muscles or attitudes may be limiting your ability to be in the world in a balanced manner. In this way Push Hands begins to make you aware of your own particular style of projecting and receiving force — a style that you may use all through your life. Further, it provides opportunities to learn how to handle force in a balanced manner.

In the first chapter, I described "aggressive, controlling behavior," a post-traumatic stress symptom, as a high degree of willingness to use physical, mental, emotional, or verbal force to achieve your goals, even when not in a survival situation. For individuals who have developed this style of behavior, it may be such a deeply ingrained way of acting that they are no longer aware that they are using projected force. Thus, in many cases what other people might judge as aggressive, controlling behavior simply seems like normal behavior to the person who is using it.

Push Hands helps you build awareness of actions that have excessive or otherwise imbalanced force in them. Now, it's important to be precise when using a word like "excessive," since it is a judgement on how much is enough and how much is too much. **Force is "excessive" when its use causes you to lose your balance.** An amount of force that is going to sabotage your ability to meet your goals drawing you off-balance is excessive. Remember, we defined balance as staying within the range of using an efficient amount of energy to achieve your goals.

Let's look at two examples of what balance has to teach from Push Hands practice. First, let's look at an individual whose life experiences have led to the development of a very aggressive style of behaving. This person wants to win and holds a desire for the other player to lose. This desire can easily displace attention from the mission of maintaining balance. The importance of maintaining the ground under one's own feet is easily forgotten. When one is thinking about "beating the other guy" as the highest goal, one is willing to sacrifice balance in order to knock this person off-balance and beat them. Although this may sometimes appear to achieve a winning position in life as well as push hands, it is a strategy that also often backfires. The use of excessive force can easily defeat your own purposes. This, of course, does not apply only to trauma survivors; it is true for all human beings.

Second, let's look at an individual whose life experience has led to the development of a very passive and non-assertive style of behaving. This person is less likely to get "hooked" by a desire to win, yet may get "stuck" in a fear-reaction when in the field of contact with another person's force. Players with this style may find it much easier to receive the force of another than to push out with their own force. When one is thinking about not engaging in opposing forces as the goal, this accommodating style may displace attention from the mission of maintaining balance also.

One use of Push Hands is to demonstrate to yourself the significance of Rebalancing. You don't need to take it on faith; if you try it you can see for yourself what happens when you push hard without regard for your own balance. If you push with great force in a way that doesn't maintain awareness of your own balance, any skilled player will get out of the way and you will move your foot position. In this case you essentially drew yourself off-balance. If you push with great force in an unbalanced manner and the other player does the same, the impact may not knock you off-balance because the forward rush of your force was slowed by the forward rush of opposing force. But if you don't know how to project your force without losing your balance, you will always be dependent on having someone or something outside of you to bounce off of. You will need someone to hit in order to feel the power of your force. With greater balance, this need is increasingly reduced.

Use of Force and Rebalancing

Aggressive, controlling behavior is really a type of behavior where we make choices about how to reach our goals that are very similar to the choice we are making when we push out with strong force in Push Hands and lose our balance. When the "fight or flight" command is giving the orders, it may be easy to get "stuck" in pushing out with great force, or losing touch with our force. Part of the healing mission where post-traumatic stress is concerned lies in gaining ability to "turn down the volume" on the intensity of this command.

It is also possible to use a style of passive-aggressive controlling force in a conscious manner in coping with threat. In this case the individual does not push out with force but instead uses force to invite the other player into an off-balance position, so they will be in a less powerful and therefore less threatening position. This is another coping style that may be used with much energy when the fight or flight alarm has sounded.

One way to effect change is to learn how to use force in a balanced way. Just as the ventilation system in an office building can be programmed to change the temperature when it moves outside the balanced range, so too can you learn more about changing your own internal "temperature." Just as an office building that has reached a 100 degree temperature will make it very stressful and uncomfortable for the people inside, so will you feel stressed and uncomfortable when the pressure inside your mind and body becomes too high. Remember, when you send the "fight or flight" command, you are telling your body to turn up the pressure. If you have learned to cope with your "unusual experiences" by using this command a great deal of the time, then you may have frequent high-pressure buildups that are very uncomfortable.

One way to practice "letting out some pressure" from a balanced position can be demonstrated through Push Hands. Stand in the Push Hands posture with knees slightly bent, head and spine erect, hips and shoulders loose, arms retracted under the shoulders at chest level with palms facing forward, fingers up. Inhale and slowly exhale. Inhale again, exhale slowly, and imagine near the end of your exhalation that you are breathing out the last bit of air through your arms, down your arms, though your hands. As you imagine this, push out your arms. When you exhale and push out with strong force, notice if your head and spine lean forward, or if they remain in their starting position. If you move your body forward as you push out with your arms, you will need to hit something solid to maintain your balance. To overcome this, exhale, push out, and keep your head and spine straight. You will be practicing pushing out your force from a balanced place. Inhale, exhale, and, near the end of your deep exhalation, push out your arms with your breath. When you become comfortable synchronizing your exhalation and arm movement, you can sense a flow of energy in motion: your energy, your force. This motion can be a satisfying release when there is pent-up pressure from anger or other unresolved tension. It can also be a useful practice for improving assertiveness skills where there is difficulty projecting force.

I have been speaking about balance because moving towards balance is a way to open up some release valves inside yourself to let out some extra pressure. You need to take some action to open these release valves, action that leads towards balance. To do this you have to know what balance is, and you have to know it not just intellectually (in your thinking mind) but as an experience, as a way to be that you can remember because you've been there. This is why it's important to cultivate balance within your own body, mind, and feelings. You are developing a "homing beacon" which can show the direction you'll want to move in when you are feeling over-stressed.

For example, when you have a tension headache, you may at first know only that you are feeling pain. Where this is the case, all you'll likely want to do is get rid of the pain. After practicing some balancing methods, however, you may become aware that you get such headaches only after a buildup of high pressure has occurred inside you. This means that you have actively tightened certain muscles in your body to cope with the stress, and these in turn have restricted blood flow and led to that headache.

If you know that all this happened before you felt the painful headache, then instead of conceiving of your task as simply making the pain go away, you might see that your task in returning to balance involves dealing with the stressful events you are reacting to and thereby reducing the tension in your muscles. In some cases, moving towards balance involves learning the skill of relaxing certain muscle groups. The specific muscles you will need to relax depend on your individual pattern of tensing and relaxing your body.

This same strategy can be applied to your thoughts. If you tend to think "paranoid" thoughts based on unreasonable fear, this will tense up your muscles as tightly as if they were reacting to a real threat. So part of what we are talking about when we talk about moving towards balance is holding to patterns of thought that do not have an unusually high fear component.

Practicing Balance: Progressive Relaxation

Knowing how to relax is an important part of moving towards balance for anyone who spends a lot of time feeling tense or anxious. For this reason I will describe a particular exercise that has proven useful in relaxing the body and calming the mind for many people. In my practice, I have taught this method to individuals while they were connected to an electromyograph. In this way an individual can measure his or her success in sending relaxation commands to the muscles. Where it is not possible to measure your muscle tension levels with electronic technology, you'll have to rely on your own internal "radar" to sense what is happening inside your body.

You can check how your muscles feel to you before and after you practice this exercise. It will actually take longer to explain this exercise than to practice it. **In this exercise, you will be taking particular actions regarding three different parts of yourself: your body, your breathing, and your thoughts.** I will discuss each action-sequence separately and then describe how to do them all at the same time.

The first part is a set of actions you can practice with your body. It is called progressive relaxation and is very simple. **In progressive relaxation, you concentrate on one muscle group at a time. First you tighten the muscles, then you "let go," that is, you relax them.** Tighten. Relax. Start with the toes: tighten, then relax. Follow these instructions for the toes, the ankles, the calf muscles, thigh muscles, butt muscles, lower back muscles, stomach muscles, the chest area, the upper back, the shoulders, the neck, the face (eyes, forehead, jaw), then the upper arms, the lower arms, and finally finish up by clenching your hands into fists, then relaxing them. Tighten. Relax. That's all there is to this first part of the exercise. Practice it at least once to get the feel.

The second part has to do with your breathing. In this exercise you will practice abdominal breathing. This will increase the oxygen coming into your body. You will breathe in through the nose and out through the mouth. When you inhale through the nose, you want to inhale fairly deeply — certainly not to the point where you feel as though your lungs will burst; merely a good, deep, and full inhalation.

Many people believe that their lungs are in their chest and that a deep inhalation means they will suck in the gut and puff out the chest. **If you look at an anatomical drawing of a human being you can see that the bottoms of the lungs actually extend down into the abdominal cavity.** This means that if you suck in your gut (pull in your stomach) while inhaling, you will block air from entering them — as if you were blowing air into one end of a balloon while pinching it at the other end. So you must practice inhaling into the bottom of your lungs to get a truly deep inhalation. Take a deep breath (inhaling through the nose) and place your hand over your solar plexus (above the naval and below the rib cage). Leave your hand about one inch out from your skin. Does this area rise slightly when you inhale? If not, you may be taking a small breath that mostly inflates only the top part of your lungs, in your chest. **Try to breathe into your abdomen so your belly inflates slightly and the skin rises to touch your hand.** This is a good sign that you are inflating your lower lungs as well.

Once you are confident that you are filling your lungs fully, you can pay attention to several other steps in abdominal breathing. The next step is to make sure that when you exhale, you do not push the air out with force, as if you were blowing out birthday candles. Instead, simply let your abdomen relax, and let the air come out with little or no force. After you inhale, your lungs are like a blown-up balloon. As you use your muscles to hold the air inside your lungs, this is similar to pinching the top of the balloon with your fingers to hold the air inside. When you exhale, simply let go as you would release the balloon with your fingers and the air will come out by itself.

To practice abdominal breathing, then, inhale through the nose into the abdomen, letting your belly rise, and then let go (exhale with no force) through the mouth. The other items I would request you pay attention to in this breathing exercise are your shoulder and jaw muscles. It is natural for your shoulders to rise slightly when you inhale and to sink as you exhale. It is natural for your jaw to lower slightly as you exhale through your mouth. If you are very tense, your jaw may stay clamped, and your shoulders may not sink at all as you exhale.

You may have to pay attention at first and give your shoulders and jaw a specific command to do these things. Now you know how to practice abdominal breathing. Inhale through the nose — let the belly expand — exhale through the mouth with no force — and let the shoulders sink and the jaw drop slightly. Try practicing it a few times to get the hang of it.

Next we will put the progressive relaxation exercise and the abdominal breathing exercise together, and do them at the same time. Progressive relaxation, remember, means tightening and then relaxing a muscle. Tighten. Relax. Two kinds of action. Abdominal breathing also has two kinds of action: Inhale. Exhale. To combine the two exercises, you time your tightening/relaxing of muscles to coordinate with your breathing in and out. Slowly tighten your toes, for example, as you slowly inhale; then slowly relax your toes as you slowly exhale.

To review what has been said, inhale slowly through your nose, letting the belly expand, while at the same time you are slowly tightening your toes. As you reach the peak of your inhalation, stop adding tension to your toe muscles. As you exhale slowly through your mouth with no force, slowly relax the tension in your toes — at the same time making sure you let your jaw and shoulders drop. Then, repeat the procedure with the next muscle group, and the next, until you've gone through them all, each time coordinating your motion so you inhale and tighten, then exhale and relax.

As I said earlier, it takes much longer to explain than to do. Going through all the muscle groups I described with this exercise should only take 3 to 5 minutes. Practice this two-part exercise to get comfortable doing the breathing and progressive relaxing at the same time.

Finally, we add a mental aspect to the exercise: visualization. While you are inhaling and exhaling and tightening and relaxing, you are also going to use your imagination to help you relax. To learn how to do this, first look at your hands, and then tighten them into fists. Next, close your eyes and picture your closed fists in your mind's eye. Then (keeping your eyes closed) open your hands, and picture this act also in your mind's eye. For the mental part of this exercise, you will be picturing the various parts of the body in this way as you are breathing in and tightening, and breathing out and relaxing. You are going to use your imagination to act upon those pictures in the mind's eye. Keep your eyes closed and practice tightening your fists as you inhale, relaxing your hands as you exhale, and seeing a picture of your hands opening and closing in your mind's eye as you clench and unclench them. Once you are comfortable with doing this, you're ready for the next step.

Close your eyes and inhale while you tighten your hands. This time, as you exhale through your mouth and relax your hands, imagine that you are also breathing out through your hands. Of course, you cannot really exhale through your hands. That doesn't matter. As you are exhaling with your eyes closed, you can imagine that you are pushing air out through your hands. In your mind's eye, watch your hands draw tighter as you inhale. As you exhale and watch your hands relax, imagine that you can see tension flowing out your hands as you exhale through them.

What does tension look like? It looks like whatever it is that you see when you do this. Some people practicing this exercise report that they imagine dark smoke coming out of their hands; others see fiery red or gray smoke. Other individuals report observing steam as from a teakettle; still others have described coiled up springs releasing their tension or hydraulic jacks returning to a state of rest. You can use any of these images or make up your own: what is important is that you somehow find a way to picture in your mind's eye that something is coming out of the body part through which you are exhaling — smoke, steam, fog, smog: anything that can represent the stored up stress in your muscles.

Many individuals have noted that as they exhale through a muscle that is actually relaxed, they see a clear-colored exhalation; as they exhale through a tight muscle, they observe a more dirty-colored exhalation. Just pick any image that works for you. When you can picture yourself "opening a release valve" in this way, you will be sending a command (from your mind, through your brain, to your muscles) that can help you relax.

Now you are ready to hear the actual instructions for the complete relaxation exercise using your mind, your body, and your breathing. Since you cannot read them and practice them at the same time, it would be helpful, while you are learning, to get another person to read them to you or to read them out loud onto a recording tape that you can play when you choose to practice. Before beginning, sit or lie down comfortably in a quiet place where you will not be interrupted. Choose a place away from the telephone if possible. Loosen any tight clothing and use the bathroom if necessary. Make sure that you pick a breathing speed that is comfortable for you, even if it doesn't exactly match the speed at which the verbal instructions are given. If the voice giving instructions speaks too slowly for you, don't hold your breath; just inhale and tighten, exhale and relax at the pace that is comfortable for you. Check inside your body with your "internal radar" system: how do your muscles feel? Take a moment to take inventory. Whoever is speaking the instructions should verbalize the following calmly, clearly, and slowly:

> Make sure you are comfortable and take a deep breath in, and out. Now, tighten your toes as you slowly inhale through your nose. Let your belly expand as you breathe in and tighten. Slowly exhale as you slowly breathe through your toes. See the tension blow right out through them. Try it again. Inhale and tighten toes and let the jaw and shoulders drop.

Next the ankles. Inhale as you tighten the ankles; breathe out right through the ankles. Again. Inhale and expand the belly; slowly breathe out with no force right through the ankles.

Now the calves of the legs. Inhale and tighten; exhale and breathe out through the calves. Let the jaw and shoulders sink as you exhale through the mouth. Once again, inhale and tighten the calves, then slowly exhale and relax.

The thigh muscles. Inhale and tighten; slowly breathe out right though the thighs. Again inhale and tighten; slowly relax and let the jaw and shoulders sink.

Next the butt muscles. Inhale and tighten; exhale and relax. Again, in through the nose and tighten, slowly breathe out and let the shoulders drop.

Lower back. Inhale and arch your lower back; breathe out through there and relax. Breathe in and tighten; exhale and watch the tension blow right out your lower back.

Stomach. Inhale and tighten; breathe out with no force. Breathe in through the nose, breathe out and let your jaw and shoulders drop.

Low back. Inhale and arch your low back; breathe out through there and relax. Breathe in and tighten; exhale and watch the tension blow right out your low back.

Stomach. Inhale and tighten; breathe out with no force. Breathe in through the nose, breathe out and let your jaw and shoulders drop.

Upper back. Inhale and flex your shoulder blades; then breathe out through your shoulder blades. Slowly inhale and tighten, then breathe out and relax.

Shoulders: inhale and hunch up your shoulders; then exhale and let them drop. Inhale and tighten; then see yourself breathing out right through the shoulders.

Now the neck. Again: in through the nose and expand the belly; breathe out with no force right through the neck. The face muscles. Inhale and tighten the eyes, jaw, and forehead; then breathe out through there and relax. Inhale and tighten, then watch the tension blow right out through your face.

Upper arms. Inhale and tighten the upper arms, then breathe out through the arms. In through the nose, then slowly exhale as you let your jaw and shoulders drop.

Lower arms and wrists: inhale and tighten, breathe out and relax. Slowly in, then slowly out.

Now we'll finish with the hands. Inhale and gather all the tension left in your body into your fists, then breathe out through your hands as you slowly relax your fingers. Again inhale and tighten, then breathe out with no force and watch the tension blow out your fingertips.

You have now completed the sequence. With practice it should take 5 minutes to move through it. Remember to sweep your body with your "internal radar" system, checking the sensations you feel there. Is there a difference before and after this exercise? Try to check this "before" and "after" each time you practice the exercise. This can help build your sensitivity to the "clues" that let you know when high pressure is building up. If you practice this relaxation sequence 3 times a day (once early, once during the day, once at night), within a few days you will very likely begin to develop a greater awareness of the ways you hold in muscle tension. I usually ask people to practice this exercise 3 times daily for 10 days. This is about the minimum time required for a fair test, to learn if it is helpful for you. **Like all relaxation methods, this technique is not magic; it's simply a way to help you become more aware of the commands your mind sends to your body.** Awareness means control; the greater your awareness, the greater the control and the easier to maintain your balance.

Rebalancing Skills and the Healing Journey

Increased ability to relax can be very helpful as you continue your self-exploration into the areas of your life that are most stressful. As you encounter these areas in your experience that most easily knock you off-balance, it is important to know what to do to help yourself stay calm and maintain ability to pay attention. As you learn to cultivate balance, you will be developing tools you can use when your "fight or flight" reflex is activated by force of habit.

Under ordinary conditions, the discipline of cultivating balance can help you experience a greater measure of peace in your daily life and an increased ability to tolerate stressful events. In the most extreme circumstances, it can be a life-saver.

The exercises I have described, like martial art forms and meditative disciplines, can be useful in helping you find your own balance by paying attention in particular ways. Although it is possible to make progress by oneself, many individuals have received great benefit from expert instruction where available, be it under the guidance of a meditation teacher, martial arts instructor, or modern therapist. It remains up to you to choose the ground where you wish to plant your feet.

5

Communicating Clear Information

Individuals with post-traumatic distress may frequently experience great difficulty in communicating clearly, but unclear communication can drive a wedge between you and your loved ones.

One very frequent cause of stress reaction is unclear communication of information. In our modern world we are frequently involved in communications containing misinformation, disinformation, and the absence of information. Many of us have forgotten how to communicate clearly and fully. For combat veterans, incest survivors, and others who have survived "unusual experiences" where communicating clearly may have been highly dangerous, reflexes may have been developed to avoid clear communication.

Communication and Threatening Situations

Sufficient exposure to danger-filled and security-conscious environments may create a reflex to withhold information not only in survival situations where life depends on it but in all situations. This type of reflex can be involved in producing stress reactions because of the relationship between unclear communications and the production of fear.

When someone asks you a direct question, for example, and you give a vague answer, the questioner may perceive you as hiding something, as not trusting them, or at the least as being unwilling to share what you know. In this situation, many individuals will experience fear — fear of you. You may have some minor reason for choosing not to communicate clearly, or you may have this reflex I am describing and not even be aware that you are withholding anything.

The other person doesn't necessarily know this. How they interpret your unclear communication may have nothing to do with your intentions — that person can have their own doubts, their own insecurities, and their own problems with self-confidence. When you communicate unclearly, they can feel fear if they perceive you to be withholding something and not know why. And then you may react to their fear, and the distance between you can be created for no other reason than unclear communication.

You will most likely not choose to communicate everything you think and feel to all people under all circumstances. In certain types of situations, however, the inability to communicate clearly can create great difficulty. In an intimate relationship, for example, suppose that your partner asks you a direct question concerning how you feel about them — and you duck the question, or at least give a vague or incomplete answer. If they are an insecure person or at least insecure concerning your feelings about them, they can use your unwillingness or inability to communicate clearly as evidence that their worst fears are true: "If they won't tell me, it must really be terrible."

The best way to safeguard against other people projecting their own worst fears into your silence is by being "straight" with them — telling them what is going on, giving them what I am calling "clear information." Remember, a person's communication can only be as clear and accurate as his or her knowledge and experience; not all questions you are asked will be questions you know the answers to. Even in this case, you can tell someone clearly that you don't have the answer to that question. If you give them the best, most accurate, and up-to-date information that you possess, you are doing the best you can. Although this will not be a priority in all circumstances, providing clear information can be essential in certain situations — such as maintaining intimacy and trust in a relationship or between friends.

Individuals with post-traumatic distress may frequently experience great difficulty in communicating clearly. When certain post-traumatic stress symptoms are experienced, for example — nightmares, recurring memories of traumatic events, or other painful occurrences connected to what happened before — a person may simply not want to talk about it. If you experience these difficulties, you may not be ready to talk about this subject, you may not want anyone else to know you are having a problem, or you may possess this reflex I have been discussing and be predisposed to withhold information.

When you do that with a loved one who knows you, who knows what you are like when you are feeling balanced, he/she may notice when you are off-balance. He/she may well think that whatever is going on inside you is somehow connected to how he/she is acting. When he/she asks you how you are doing, and you tell him/her everything is fine — well, if he/she can see that everything is not fine, then he/she may wonder what he/she has done to cause the trouble.

In this way, **your unclear communication can drive a wedge between you and your loved ones, because it can make them doubt their own perceptions.** If they notice when you are off-balance, and you choose not to tell them, they either have to believe you are withholding or that in some way what they are seeing is inaccurate — which can undermine their trust in their own perceptions.

Especially in intimate relationships, giving unclear information can cause the recipient to feel "crazy" or otherwise off-balance. In relations that are important, then, you will reduce stress reactions for yourself and your intimate others by cultivating the ability to communicate openly, honestly, and clearly.

Practicing Clear Communication: "Checking In"

Communicating clear information isn't always easy. Sometimes we can intend to communicate clearly and muck it up anyway. For example, we can communicate a message whose meaning is very clear to us but makes no sense at all to the other person; or worse yet, makes a different kind of sense than what we intended. **Communicating clear information involves not only speaking your mind but also making sure that the message you intend to convey is the message the other person receives.** Another way to say this is that we must check to make sure both people are speaking the same language. I call this type of making sure about the reception of your broadcasts "checking in"; we can check with the other person to make sure our messages have been understood and, of course, their messages too.

Let me give an example. Suppose in an intimate relationship one partner (A) comes home from work, and the other partner (B) initiates a conversation. B has been lonely and wants to be reassured that A cares for her. What B actually says, however, is: "We hardly spend any time together anymore. Sometimes I wonder if you're avoiding me."

What B really wanted to know was if A still loved her and valued B's friendship. But B did not ask this question in a clear way. A, who was feeling overworked, heard a very different question than the one B intended to ask. A heard B asking why A was not giving B what B needs ("we hardly spend time together") and felt as if this was criticism. A did not know B was asking for reassurance; A heard B telling A that A was doing something wrong. And so A's defensive response: "I'm doing the best I can!" is not a response to the real question B was asking — ("Do you love me?").

Now B, who really believes that it was clearly asked if A loves B and that A understood this question, hears A's response — "I'm doing the best I can!" — as if it were a response to B's question about whether or not A loves B. To B's ears, A's reply makes it sound as if it's really a tough effort for A to love B. When B hears A's reply, B interprets the message as "Don't ask me for anything more." B's worst fear is realized, B believes: all B is asking for is love and A will not give it.

These people are not communicating on the same wavelength, and it is easy to see how fear can gain hold in both of them. Not because of any real disagreement between the participants, but because they didn't take the time to make sure that their communications were clear. Because both these people had some insecurity and some fear concerning their status with each other, they immediately filled in the unknowns in the unclear communications with their worst fears.

To defuse this type of misunderstanding, it is necessary to practice "checking in" with the other person, which means taking responsibility for making sure that the message transmitted and the message received are in fact the same. Going back to our example, either party could have taken responsibility to "check in" and thereby avoid misunderstanding. A — when first hearing B's initial question — could have asked for further clarification. Instead of being certain that A was under attack, A could have "checked in" by asking for more words to help describe the meaning intended: "are you telling me I'm doing something wrong?" or "what exactly are you asking me?" In this way he could have given B more opportunity to become clear in communicating B's essential question. Instead of reacting to the negative message that A believed he heard, A could have gathered further information which would have shown that A was interpreting the message incorrectly.

In the same way, B also had opportunity to practice the skill of "checking in." When A responded to B by saying "I'm doing the best I can!," B could also "check in" to make sure that the message B received was the same as the one intended: "Are you saying you don't care about me?" or "what do you mean by that?"

Sometimes we will mishear others in line with our hidden desires (what we want to hear); other times what we hear may be distorted by our hidden fears. In either case, exercising the skill of "checking in" during important communications will help minimize confusion and increase our certainty that the meaning we heard is the meaning that's really there.

Respectful Communication

In this discussion on clear communication I would also like to mention the concept of respectful communication. As I am using the term, "respectful communication" refers not so much to the content of what is said, but more to a particular process by which information is transmitted. In attempting to communicate respectfully, a person is choosing to do the best they can to find ways to disseminate information that are least threatening to the listener(s). This means that what gets said is no more important than finding ways to say it that create a minimum of "nonpeace" between communicator and listener, ways that acknowledge that some communications can stimulate the "fight or flight" alarm for some listeners. To create safety in communicating, and especially in communicating about emotionally charged subjects, take responsibility for your feelings, perceptions, and interpretations rather than communicating them as "the truth." Be careful to fully claim your judgements and criticisms of others with qualifying phases like "It looks to me like. . ." or "I feel that. . .," or any other such form that acknowledges that you are aware that what you are communicating belongs to you, the communicator. It is much more likely that you will communicate a sense of attack if you say "You are terrible" rather than "I feel like I'm seeing something terrible in you," because in the first statement there is no implied permission allowing another point of view. Either I accept I am terrible, or I have to reject you, the communicator, and both may be experienced as nonpeaceful alternatives. In the latter phrasing, there is at least recognition that this sense of terribleness is an opinion of the communicator, and the listener has received the basic human freedom to disagree. This may seem like a minor shift, but communicating in ways that allow others to view matters differently can go a long way towards defusing fear reactions and promoting mutual respect.

Disrespectful Communication

I have been speaking up to this point about unintentional confusion in communicating; sometimes unclear communicating is quite intentional. One example is what I call the "I don't know" reflex. We may use it when we are angry or otherwise feeling less than generous about sharing what we know. This is a passive-aggressive style of communicating, which means we can be aggressive without admitting it and without appearing aggressive on the surface.

Withholding information by acting like you don't have it is a way to hold the upper ground and keep the other person in a confused, less powerful position. Whatever the surface denial may sound like (and there are many variations), it is actually quite an aggressive communication style because of its highly unclear information content. The "I don't know" reflex is observable in action by the complete absence of clear information:

Q. What would you like for breakfast?
A. I don't know.
Q. How about corn flakes or eggs?
A. I don't care.
Q. Want some orange juice?
A. Doesn't matter.
Q. Are you awake yet?
A. I don't know.

The "I don't know" style is a way to avoid being present without taking responsibility for not being present. It leaves the other person in an unclear position, and they may become frightened if they don't understand why you are unwilling to transmit clear information. **Clear information transmission becomes easier as you take responsibility for your communications.** Remember that silence is another form of communication. However you respond is filled with communicative information — whether you respond fully, partially, in silence, or in withdrawal.

During the communications in which you choose to have the greatest trust and intimacy, remember that unclear communication breeds fear. Honest and clear information dispels fear. If you are having difficulties in being understood by others, look to the quality of your communications. Any tensions may have at least as much to do with the different languages you speak as with material differences of substance. Learning to practice clear communication, especially with loved ones, can save you pain and confusion. This is emphatically true for trauma survivors, who may have developed a withholding communication style during life events that held real danger.

Trust, Fear, and Respectful Communication

Another area of communication that has a good deal to do with the production of stress reactions is the area of communicating criticism and appreciation. **If you are using a communication style developed in a survival environment, you may have developed special priorities concerning the things you choose to talk about.** You may, for example, be much more likely to speak critical thoughts than appreciative thoughts. Or, conversely, you may be more willing to voice your appreciative thoughts and withhold your critical thoughts. It depends on individual experience, and in this is similar to the Push Hands exercise where some individuals can push out with great force but do not know how to bend, while others can receive force quite easily, but do not know how to push with their force.

In a combat environment, for example, it might be considered a sign of good intentions if you inform someone who is doing something less effectively than possible, because without knowledge of how to do things correctly, they may not be able to survive.

In a dysfunctional, violent family, on the other hand, voicing critical thoughts might be met with an immediate increase in danger, while safety may be found only in speaking appreciative thoughts. And so in this very different type of situation one may develop a very different communication style.

Although these styles may be valuable for survival efficiency in dangerous circumstances, they can also create stress in social situations. Those who do not understand these communication styles may, at one extreme, not understand when you criticize them more frequently than you appreciate them and may feel picked on, abused, and disrespected. At the other extreme, others may get no clues at all from your feedback when they do something "not okay" if you cannot voice your critical thoughts yet may feel some distance without the essential information they need to understand and may therefore also feel disrespected.

If you are carrying excessive anger, verbal criticism may also be a method you use to ventilate some of the pressure of that anger. When you ventilate in this manner in the direction of innocent bystanders, however, you may damage your relationships unintentionally. When you have important criticism to relay to someone, you will do well to pick the spots to express your feelings by choosing the moments when you are experiencing your greatest balance. Learning this skill of choosing the right moment is another important communication choice acting in service of fear reduction.

To this point I have mostly been discussing the sending of critical and appreciative communications. It is equally important to pay attention to your style of receiving these types of communications. Can you accept criticism from others without experiencing strong stress reactions? How about appreciation? If either critical or appreciative communications about you consistently knock you off-balance, then you may need to ask just what it is that you are finding threatening in such communications. This task may be particularly important where post-traumatic distress is present, because survivors may have impairments in ability to listen to any information that sounds like, feels like, or otherwise reminds them of previous traumatic events. Earlier I discussed the phenomenon of dissociation as an inability to stay present with what is happening now. Threatening communications can be major triggers causing dissociative reactions. What this means is that if you find an area in your experience where there is a consistent inability to listen, this may be a clue that stress reaction and/or dissociation is taking place. This is another way to recognize fear as an obstacle to clear communication.

Practicing Clear Communication:
Criticism and Appreciation

One good exercise for working on developing communication skills is the "Appreciation Sandwich" exercise. The guidelines for this exercise are that two people agree to take turns in the role of "speaker" and "listener." The speaker will make three statements about the other person. The first statement must be an appreciative statement completing this sentence: "I value you because. . . ." The second statement is a critical statement completing this sentence: "I'm having problems with your way of. . . ." The third statement is again an appreciative statement: "I value you because. . . ."

The task of the speaker during this exercise is to communicate as clearly as possible, to stay within the guidelines without elaborations, and to choose statements that are both sincere and relevant to the relationship. The listener's task is to sit quietly, without speaking or gesturing, and to listen actively to all that is communicated. Then the roles are reversed, and the same process is repeated in the opposite direction. In this way, individuals can practice both expressing and receiving communications related to both criticism and appreciation.

The "appreciation sandwich" exercise can be extended into a communication reception exercise for those who wish to practice the skill of "checking in" about messages sent and messages received. After the basic exercise is completed, each person can take a turn "checking in" by stating what they heard when the other person made their three statements to make sure that the critical and appreciative messages intended were the same as the ones received. Two individuals can practice this exercise alone; however, it is important to practice the exercise without giving voice to any defensive reactions that may occur about the critical statements received.

When you are honestly stating your feelings and the other person is doing the same, you are both "right" — even if you disagree completely. Where you are interested in allowing clear communications to occur, you must allow the other person to have their feelings — even if you are convinced they are ignorant, illogical, or otherwise out-of-touch with reality. If you fall into the trap of invalidating the other person by trying to argue them out of their human right to feel as they do, you will sabotage the communication. In a sense, this strategy is identical to that described for playing Push

Hands. When you are communicating clearly in this manner, you will be able to push out your (verbal) force and receive that of others without losing balance.

If in practice you and your partner find you cannot follow the basic ground rules of this exercise, it may be necessary to use a "referee." A trained therapist or at least a good listener can help you in practicing accurate listening and developing the skill of effectively communicating clear information. With enhanced communication skill you can act more effectively in pursuing your social goals and maintaining balance in the face of unclear information transmitted by others. Perhaps best of all, communicating clearly will enable you to experience the power of your voice both in service of constructive change (criticism) or in direct expression of caring (appreciation).

6

Reinforcing the Immune System

The "combat readiness" of your immune system depends in part on what you are thinking about, what you are feeling, and the foods and other substances you take into your body.

We will now look at some of the reasons it may be important for you to take action to strengthen your immune system. There is a relationship between high stress and immune function (how well or poorly your immune system is working): **Exposure to prolonged high stress may weaken your immune strength.** Under normal conditions, we are constantly exposed to a barrage of germs, bacteria, and exotic life-forms, that under certain circumstances, can grow at an imbalanced rate inside our bodies, giving rise to diseases.

Balance, Stress, and Immune Function

The various "troops" of our immune system that man our "shore defenses" and resist those invading germs are usually adequate to prevent their establishing beachheads in our bodies. The immune system acts to maintain various kinds of balance. It sends out scouts patrolling the chemical "soup" of our liquid tissues, engages in combat where it contacts hostile life-forms, and sends reports to headquarters (the unconscious brain) about the situation in the field. In performing all these tasks, the immune system is acting in service of its primary mission, which is to maintain a complicated pattern of balance in the "brew" of our life-juices. It is the field soldier in our body's chain of command: when the warriors are working in harmony, the body has considerable power to defend itself from invaders.

Recent research has shown that our mental functioning has some influence on the chemical balance of the immune system. This means that when the "orders from headquarters" are contradictory, unclear, and outright unreasonable, the "soldiers in the field" are going to have a hard time defending the integrity of the body. If the "orders" received by the immune system are garbled by static from anywhere in the body/mind/brain communication system, then the "field commanders" of the immune system may not know enough about the total situation to make the right tactical decisions. Troop strength may fall, supplies may run low, positions may get overrun. Resistance to outside invaders may decline, or certain elements of the defensive system may mutiny and grow in an imbalanced way.

It is becoming increasingly clear that many diseases gain a beachhead within the body only after certain immune defenses have been knocked out of commission (out of balance). This is why it is so important to keep immune defenses well-nourished and as adaptable and sensitive to change as possible. On the basis of well-established research, it can be argued that the "combat readiness" of your body's immune system depends in part on what you are thinking about, what you are feeling, and the foods and other substances you burn as fuels. In discussing the idea of "reinforcing the immune system," I am basically trying to pass on some information about simple methods available to anyone who chooses to send some supplies to the front lines in support of the body's effort to maintain health.

The types of changes in the body that are associated with high stress — especially prolonged high stress — limit the power of the immune system's defenses. We still do not understand all the reasons why this is true, but there is sufficient evidence to know that high stress and weak immune functions are connected.

Under prolonged high stress, you are more likely to be susceptible to a variety of viruses, cancers, other infectious diseases, autoimmune diseases (where the "foot soldiers" of the immune system start fighting among themselves), and allergies. The whole picture is even more complicated when we discuss immune systems that have not only experienced prolonged stress but also have been highly exposed to toxic chemicals. **Toxic chemicals have also been implicated in weakening the power of the immune system.**

Chemical Poisoning, Stress, and Immune Function

I first began paying attention to these relationships in my work with Vietnam veterans. With millions of gallons of Agents Orange, Blue, White, etc. sprayed on Vietnam during that war, a large number of Vietnam veterans were exposed to such toxic chemicals. Some of those who received the most severe exposures are no longer living; this tragedy is one part of the ugly legacy of the aftermath of the war. We will probably never be certain of all the Vietnam-exposure health effects. It is very difficult for most veterans to measure exactly what their exposure was, since everyone who drank the water, breathed the air, and ate the food wherever these chemicals were used in Southeast Asia received at least some exposure not only to Agent Orange and its most lethal component (2,3,7,8 TCDD-dioxin) but also to a variety of other compounds as well. However, this type of problem is by no means limited to veterans; their experience merely preceded what is now an increasingly generalized exposure in the industrialized, chemical-laden modern world. A 1986 study of one thousand North American nursing mothers, for example, found that almost all breast milk samples contained some amount of 2,3,7,8 TCDD-dioxin. This is one of many indications that all of us living in modern industrialized countries are at increased risk from toxic chemical assaults that may be a factor in our health.

Our government has been very slow to acknowledge the toxic health effects of these chemicals — primarily for political and economic reasons. Given the poor quality of record keeping and the multiple substances to which we are potentially exposed, it may not be possible to measure just how much any particular exposure has impacted your health. Our task here is not to prove that any particular exposure was responsible for any problems you may have now, or to prove that anything else was responsible for your current difficulties. The task is to consider what the healing possibilities are now.

When we are talking about the immune system, there are certain "clues" to how well your immune system is functioning. Some of these "clues" are general signs such as your susceptibility to common colds, allergies, or temperature shifts. Other clues relate to specific symptoms associated with exposure to specific chemicals. Here I will discuss only exposure to dioxin. One form of dioxin (there are approximately 75 varieties) is the most lethal constituent in one of the two ingredients in Agent Orange, 2,4,5,T herbicide. Dioxin generally, and especially this particular form of dioxin (2,3,7,8 TCDD-dioxin), has been implicated in diminishing the strength of various components of the immune response in humans and other animals. For our purposes here I will not review all the chemical changes and blood alterations that have been demonstrated to correlate with dioxin exposure; I will only discuss those symptoms of exposure that are easy for nonmedical people to observe themselves.

One characteristic symptom of dioxin poisoning (it's most likely to show up in heavily exposed people) is called chloracne, a particular kind of skin rash. See figure 5 for an accurate identification of what chloracne looks like. If you now have or have had a skin rash that looks like this, this may be a "clue" that your immune system needs some reinforcing. This is especially true if you first got this rash following exposure to toxic chemicals (in Vietnam or anywhere else) and experience some other general symptoms.

Chemical exposure has caused a weakening of the body's defenses for many individuals in industrialized nations. In recent years, as more and more doctors have, over time, observed the effects of strong chemicals on more and more of their patients, a new way of talking about this kind of imbalance has evolved. Medical jargon and legal rulings in several states now refer to "chemical sensitivity disorder" or "chemically induced immune dysregulation syndrome" to acknowledge the kinds of imbalances that show up in human immune systems that have been exposed to toxic chemicals.

Not surprisingly, the "laundry list" of symptoms observed in those poisoned by a wide variety of chemicals here in America is quite similar to the "laundry list" of physical disease symptoms reported by heavily exposed Vietnam veterans. A short version of these lists would include chloracne, liver disorders, kidney disorders, neurological disorders, respiratory disorders, birth defects (especially cleft lip, cleft palate, and spina bifida), auto-immune diseases (such as multiple sclerosis, rheumatoid arthritis, and lupus erythematosus), and diseases caused by viral agents (such as cancers). Viral agents can infiltrate the body's defense system with greater ease in individuals who have acquired an immune deficiency through any of several pathways, including toxic chemical exposures.

One key symptom of "chemical sensitivity disorder" — which includes the weakened immune symptoms I just described — is increased reactivity upon exposure to toxic environments. Stress and anxiety reactions can occur upon exposure, as well as headaches, allergic reactions, general arousal, and in general worsening of preexisting disease symptoms.

In some cases relatively mild chemical exposures can elicit strong reactions. For example, four veterans with moderate to severe chloracne and a history of toxic chemical exposure reported similar reactions when they walked past a perfume counter in a department store: elevated anxiety, difficulty breathing, headaches, and an initial activation of their "fight or flight" reflex (general quarters sounding off). This type of reaction might occur from a variety of different chemical exposures, such as to a freshly painted room, or to thick rushhour traffic. These exposed people realized that when they had this type of reaction, their bodies were sending them messages: the systems that kept their bodies balanced were being overloaded.

When we talk about chemical sensitivity disorder, essentially what we are saying is that our immune systems, when weakened by exposure to toxic chemicals, have lost some ability to tolerate stress. Whereas before it had a larger capability to fight off and flush out poisons and still maintain balance, now the same amount of poison is more than it can handle. Smaller amounts of toxic exposure are all the system can take. **Where immune function is seriously weakened, the body cannot tolerate any chemical exposure without losing balance.**

Individuals with chemical sensitivity disorder, then, have a greater need to continually reinforce the immune system in order to maintain balance and deal with the stresses of modern-day life. This can be life-saving information if you are having stress reactions that are related to your "unusual experiences" and are also compounded by your inability to tolerate toxic environments.

Three coffee-drinking veterans with chemical sensitivity disorder reported that they experienced stress reactions when they drank coffee from styrofoam cups. These men noted that they did not experience stress reactions if they drank coffee from non-styrofoam cups. I relate this observation as an example that suggests that there are many actions that are considered "normal" and "not harmful" by the great majority of Americans that may in fact be directly involved in causing some reactions that are very uncomfortable for you. **If you do have serious immune imbalance, it is going to interact with any post-traumatic stress-related imbalances that are also present.**

If you have chloracne, if you display signs of chemical sensitivity disorder, and if you have a history of toxic chemical exposure, you need to be honest with yourself about observing these imbalances. Only then will you choose to take any actions that may reinforce your immune strength.

Strengthening Immune Function: A New Frontier

Methods for immune enhancement are still very controversial. Among scientists, a new medical field is being created called (don't worry, you won't be tested on pronunciation) psychoneuroimmunology (PNI) or psychoneuroimmunoendocrinology (PNIE). Psycho=the mind, neuro=the nervous system, immuno=the immune system, and endocrinology=the glandular system that produces hormones. PNIE studies how the mind, the brain and the rest of the nervous system, the immune system, and the endocrine glands communicate and work together to create balance and imbalance in the body. PNIE ask questions about how our minds, our immune strength, our nerves, and our hormones all influence each other. What happens in the immune system that influences mind, nerves, glands? What happens in the mind that influences nerves, immune strength, and glands?

Since these types of holistic questions are so new for modern science, there is still a long way to go. We do know that positive, calming, and tranquil thoughts have in some cases been shown to reiforce the immune system. We also know that prolonged high stress from a variety of causes is associated with stimulating activities in the immune system that are equivalent to reducing troop strength among the immune system's "grunts" in the field. These facts are one of the reasons I keep emphasizing the importance of cultivating balance in maintaining health.

In my work with trauma survivors with multiple physical problems as well as trauma-related difficulties, it is often very difficult to know with certainty just how big a role toxic chemical exposure is playing in causing or promoting the difficulties that any particular individual is experiencing. Much of the available research on the subject is misleading or, at best, difficult to interpret. If you cannot rely on the medical literature (most of which was not written by scientists who have studied PNIE) to supply clear information about the relationships between toxic exposure, stress, and distress, who else knows about such things? Who else has paid attention? Who else has a track record in studying what can be done to help humans cope with the chronic effects of exposure to poisons?

Purification by Sweating: A Natural Method

In seeking answers to these questions, I began to consider the available alternatives to simply making believe toxic chemical problems weren't there or that nothing helpful could be done for exposed individuals. One of the first things I noticed was the research on immune strength related to nutrition. The foods we take in as fuel are very important in reinforcing or weakening the immune system. You need to eat the right foods and eat them regularly.

There is no one recognized formula for the "right" diet; every individual has some variations in their needs. However, we all need a variety of basic dietary vitamins and minerals. A good rule of thumb is to include a high percentage of fresh food and limit the intake of refined and processed foods in your diet. Emphasis on fruits and vegetables and de-emphasis on red meats, sugars, and fats are all associated with lower cancer rates and other clues pointing towards healthy immune function.

In recent years there have been increased reports of individuals with extreme immune weakness regaining considerable immune balance through dietary changes alone. If you eat mostly processed foods, if you frequently do not eat for days at a time, or if your body is so weakened that it is unable to extract nutrients from the foods you eat, you will need to take a hard look at your diet if you seriously choose to strengthen your immune responses.

Heavy alcohol consumption, tobacco smoking, and controlled substance use have also been implicated in immune suppression imbalances. Addictions (to foods and other substances) are always touchy subjects. Although I'd like to avoid being accused of over-simplifying the issues by telling anybody to "just say no," suffice it to say that if your addictions gain control of you, then you may lose control of your immune defenses as well as creating other imbalances. To reinforce your immune system, increase the number of good choices about what you feed yourself both in the substances you eat and drink and the thoughts you take in from your environment. Thoughts that are most vital and alive can strengthen you.

One pioneering inquiry can be found in the research of Z. Gard, a physician from Missouri. Dr. Gard was a U.S. Public Health Service physician who observed the health effects of toxic chemicals on people from Times Beach, Missouri. Times Beach is among the worst dioxin-contaminated sites in the U.S. It was so severely poisoned that the U.S. government bought the entire town and condemned it. The citizens of Times Beach were exposed to 2, 3,7,8 TCDD-dioxin — the same stuff found in Agent Orange.

Dr. Gard, in seeking answers as to how to help chemical poisoning victims, established a chemical detoxification facility in San Diego, California. His method of treatment uses pure food, pure water, pure air, and a pure natural environment as well as intensive sweating through exposure to heat in a sauna. Patients may sweat up to several hours a day and are closely monitored by medical staff to insure that vital signs do not diverge from safe limits. Dr. Gard measured the serum levels of poison victims before and after various kinds of toxic chemicals emigrated out of the body through perspiration. These chemicals were indeed present in the perspiration excreted from the body. So, we know there is at least one method to begin to get toxic chemicals moving out of the body. Unfortunately, such methods are not yet widely available and are also quite expensive. These expenses are not covered by most private insurance companies, and they are definitely not authorized for payment by the federal government, which fears (rightly so) multibillion dollar liabilities if this type of thinking is acknowledged.

In searching for simple methods of treatment of chemical poisoning that are relatively inexpensive, I remembered the native American sweat lodge ceremony, a very ancient method of cleansing. I had some information about these ceremonies and thought that healing methods like this might provide a way to help people detoxify. It is very simple, can be done in an isolated setting without extensive medical facilities, and is virtually cost free. A traditional native American sweat lodge ceremony is a multi-dimensional ritual, which means it involves more than just the physical aspect of heating the body. I will not be describing the use of the traditional native American sweat ceremony here because I am not a native American medicine person empowered or trained to do so. I will simply report my observations of the common elements that occur when humans participate in taking a sweat, and why these occurrences may have healing value.*

---

*For information about traditional Native American sweat ceremonies, contact your local Native American medicine man or woman.

In my practice I borrow from the basic method at the core of the native American sweat procedure. This process involves using earth, in the form of igneous rocks (those of volcanic origin), and storing fire inside the earth by heating the rocks in a wood fire. Next, water is poured upon the rocks (earth-with-fire-inside) in the enclosed space of the sweat "lodge" or hut. When this is done, the heat is transferred to the water and dispersed through the air, in the form of steam. Earth, fire, air, and water, in a natural setting. These are basic elements in a sweat procedure.

Focusing attention upon the power and simplicity of these basic elements is useful in helping cleanse the body, mind, and spirit. **The sweat is a purification ceremony, "boiling things down" until only the essential is left.** Back to basics. I had first learned of sweats in association with Vietnam veterans through the work of a counseling group in Port Angeles, Washington. They had reported some beneficial effects in helping veterans participate in such cleansing experiences using sweat ceremonies. As I began to offer sweats in Olympia — we called them "vet sweats" — on a regular basis, I saw that sweats were helpful in more ways than I had imagined.

The basic experience of "taking a sweat" involves several phases of action. These can be stated as:

1. Coming together
2. Returning to nature
3. Heating the rocks (waiting)
4. Accepting the heat
5. Getting purified
6. Coming out
7. Returning to balance

In choosing to take a sweat, you are choosing to work on purification. This is a psychological shift in that you take some control by cleansing the body. As you approach the sweat site, you are "taking a time out" of your daily routine. You are also choosing to participate in a group activity with a healing intention. In "vet sweats" where many participants disliked group activities, this choice was unusual and helped stretch old reflexes.

Sweat sites — best chosen in isolated natural settings near moving water — allow an opportunity to pay attention to natural beauty. There is time to do this, a rarity in our "hurry-up" modern world. There is a quiet period while the heat of the fire is transferred to the rocks. This process will take as long as it takes: you cannot make it go faster than its natural speed. For some, this is a good reminder about patience.

When in the sweat lodge — a small dark space reminiscent to many Vietnam veterans of a "hooch" — many individuals experience a brief claustrophobia or other discomfort upon first exposure to intense heat. Learning to tolerate this discomfort, learning to let it be there and accepting its presence in service of a higher goal (cleansing yourself) requires an attitude we could call the "attitude of allowing." When you adopt this attitude in your mind, you are acknowledging your discomfort to yourself and choosing to stay present.

As you accept the heat in the sweat and tolerate the discomfort, the experience changes. As you "get cooked" by the heat, your lungs and sinuses will open, you will sweat profusely, and your heart may beat rapidly. Your attention may shift away from distracting worldly problems and focus on the intense presence in the here-and-now of fire, air, earth, and water.

Eventually, the heat will be gone or you will reach your limit, and exit the sweat lodge. At this point you may feel great exhilaration — you may also feel extremely dizzy. Your highly heated and scantily clad body will not feel cold, at first, even if it is quite chilly outside. Your muscles will likely feel profoundly relaxed, and breathing deeply may require less effort than usual.

If you are dizzy, it should pass in a few minutes as your system returns to balance. **According to the ancient medicine practitioners, the sweat discharges the physical poisons from the body, poisonous thoughts from the mind, and poisonous blight from the soul.** There is unquestionably a deeply relaxing effect in this return to balance, even for individuals who have great difficulty in relaxing.

The directions for using a small, highly mobile, and low budget sweating facility are as follows. What you need to start is a pile of igneous rocks, some firewood, a 12' x 12' plastic tarp, a shovel, a gallon jug of water, and some pliable branches 6' in length. Igneous rocks are rocks that were heated in some type of volcanic heat. It's very important to get that kind of rock, because any rock with a high water content (like river rocks) can blow up when heated or when water is poured on them. Your sweat site may be in an area where volcanic rocks are available on the ground; if not you'll have to find them somewhere else and bring them along. Smaller rocks are easier to heat, so try and use rocks that are grapefruit-sized or smaller. A dozen rocks that size should be enough to get you started.

Once you have some rocks, you'll need to choose a sweat site. Ideally, sweat sites should be located next to moving water. Moving water is a powerful cleansing force: when a pool is muddy and stagnant, it can be cleansed by the flow of moving water. When we are participating in this type of cleansing and purifying experience, moving water is a very powerful and wordless reminder that this natural motion of life is a way to clean the muddy pools inside ourselves.

In my observations of sweating methods, choosing a site next to moving water adds an important dimension to the experience. Whether this is due to a high presence of negative ions at such places, immediate access to using the cool water after sweating, the soothing sounds of the water, or to other influences I don't know. I can only report that choosing a site by moving water increases the healing power of the experience; perhaps this needs to be experienced to be understood. Try it both ways and draw your own conclusions.

Once you have chosen a sweat site and acquired rocks, you'll also need some tree branches or shoots from a species that is flexible. Willow species are widely used by native peoples and widely distributed in North America. I would suggest using these if you can find them. If not, find branches or shoots of some woody plant that grows near the sweat site. Find relatively straight branches or shoots 6' high. The smaller the branch thickness, the easier to build this type of portable sweat.

Six branches are enough to build a fairly sturdy sweat lodge. Dig six holes in the ground in a circle with a diameter of 6' to 8'. Dig the holes deep enough that they will hold the branches in place when you insert them into the holes (larger end at the bottom). Dig a hole in the center of the circle about 6" deep. Bend the tops together in the center of the circle to form a dome-shaped structure (see figure 6). Place a covering over the structure and seal the edges to make the bottom airtight.

Buffalo hides and other animal skins are the traditional sweat lodge coverings; unfortunately, the supply is very short these days. You can use a sheet of 3 mil black plastic — 12' by 12' or larger — or any other material that will retain heat in the lodge. This is the only essential item among the necessary materials that might cost you some money ($5 to $10) if you don't have anything handy.

Place the rocks near a fire pit. Choose half a dozen or more apple to grapefruit-sized rocks for each round of sweating. You may want to work up to doing more than one round at each sweat. You'll need to heat as many rocks as it takes until you feel well sweated. This can vary tremendously for individuals, and you will have to find your own limits. I would suggest that for most people, one round of 6 or 7 grapefruit-sized rocks is plenty for the first time. Heat enough rocks for one or two rounds at a time. If you try to heat too many rocks at once without first sufficiently building your supply of hot coals, you might choke off your fire. Choose a fire site that is safe and nondestructive to the environment. You'll need a pretty good blaze to heat the rocks, so make sure you've got the ability to control any sparks and ashes that might get wind blown towards the local ground cover. Keep water and shovel close at hand and follow local fire regulations: it is definitely not enjoyable to have confrontations with forest rangers or local police while preparing a sweat.

Build up a decent supply of hot coals in your fire before you add any rocks. This will help reduce the chance of choking the fire when you do add rocks. Add 2 or 3 rocks, then a layer of wood, then more rocks, more wood, and so on. Keep your fire good and hot for one to two hours, depending on weather, the quality of the wood, and how seriously you wish to sweat.

When the rocks are hot, use a shovel or a pair of tongs (two stout sticks will work if you don't have anything else) to pick the rocks out of the fire. They should be glowing hot. Knock any hot coals off the rocks; these can burn for quite a while and in the enclosed lodge may create a lot of smoke. Place the hot rocks in the pit in the center of the lodge.

Remove clothing, watches, and jewelry and enter the lodge. Remember especially to remove watches, as the heat may damage them. You can wear swimsuits or shorts if you prefer. If you do wear clothing during a sweat, make sure you wash it thoroughly afterwards as it may become soaked with body toxins released through your sweat. Make sure as you enter the lodge not to touch the hot rocks in the middle; they can cause serious burns.

Someone who is familiar with the sweat should enter first and make sure that everyone entering is adequately protected from touching the rocks. Using a flashlight or candle at this point may be helpful as there is very poor lighting inside, especially if the sweat is at night. You will need a gallon container of water and a cup or ladle to pour the water onto the rocks.

You may also choose to use some medicinal herbs — this is optional. Sage, eucalyptus, and pine have all been used as sweat herbs. Herbs are placed on the hot rocks during the sweat. They release their essential properties into the steam that is produced, and this provides a direct method to deliver the healing agents of the plants into the body. Some herbs help relax the muscles, some help open the sinuses and lungs, and others simply smell pleasant.

Once the people and supplies are inside, seal the entrance and sit facing the center where the rocks are in the pit. Very slowly, at first, whoever is designated as the watertender sprinkles a few drops upon the rocks. At this point in a traditional ceremony, some time might be spent praying, chanting, singing, or otherwise preparing for the cleansing heat to come. For current purposes it is sufficient to remind yourself — in whatever way is most natural for you — why you have chosen to be present for this cleansing experience. Paying attention in this way may help you to maintain your balance as you receive the heat. Continue adding water to the rocks very slowly, raising the temperature gradually to a level where sweat is produced. Once the surface glow of the rocks is diminished, you can begin to sprinkle some herbs on the rocks as you continue to add water. If you use herbs too soon, they will burn and produce smoke, making it very difficult to breathe.

Repeat this process of adding water, sprinkling herbs, and receiving heat until the heat is gone from the rocks or until someone has experienced as much heat as can be tolerated. If anyone says they need to leave, let them out immediately. Everyone has his own limit and should not be criticized for reaching it sooner than someone else's expectations allowed. Other participants who wish to complete the round can reseal the entrance and continue.

It is worth emphasizing that many trauma survivors have been conditioned to tolerate unusually high discomfort/pain thresholds due to previous experience and may therefore remain in the sweat environment beyond a point that is medically sound. Each individual should ideally monitor his or her own breathing and heart rate and choose to leave when these move near the edge of acceptable limits. In recognition that many individuals may not make good choices regarding these limits, however, it is advised that sweat facilitators practice "checking in" and observation of participants to insure safety.

When you come out of the lodge, you may feel extremely dizzy. Your body has been heated to a much higher temperature than that to which it is accustomed, and this has likely created a temporary imbalance. At this point you may simply wish to sit or lie quietly for a few moments until your equilibrium returns. Then you can expose your body to another somewhat extreme temperature shift by jumping into the moving water nearby.

This exposure to cool water following exposure to heat is a fairly severe shift and may not be a wise choice for everyone. On your first sweat, you might try dipping your feet in the water or wrapping a towel soaked in cool water around your head. Again, you will have to judge your limit by sensing your state at the time.

Individuals with high blood pressure or heart irregularities, as well as participants with bullet fragments, shrapnel, or other metal in their bodies should wait several minutes after coming out of the sweat before entering cool water. Too sudden a change may cause pain or overly stress the heart and blood vessels.

If a little cool water feels good, you can try a little more. When you are ready, you can immerse your whole body in the cool waters. If you choose to do so, you can repeat the entire sweat procedure.

If you do not jump in the cool water following a sweat, take a shower at your earliest opportunity. The sweat released during the cleansing process may be very toxic as it is breaking down bodily poisons stored in your body's fatty tissues and excreting them through your sweat.

After the sweat, it is a good idea to take several quiet minutes around the fire to enjoy the stillness, while your body is returning to a balanced temperature. At this point it is likely that your muscles will be more relaxed, your thoughts less anxious, and that your contact with the basic elements will generally increase your pleasure in being alive. It may indeed feel very good to be alive. This feeling of well-being is a very important "homing beacon" in efforts to find your place of balance. It represents an attitude towards living that is at the core of spiritual renewal.

The more we talk about such things, however, the further away we get from being there. Suffice it to say that the sweat procedure helps to remind us of primordial simplicity by focusing attention on that which is common to all of us — like fire, air, earth, and water. For people who have had a large dose of the uglier aspects of living and the experience of war, this method may be useful in bringing attention back towards other aspects of human reality: natural simplicity and the experience of peace. Fire, air, earth, and water. Try it and see for yourself.

Sweats, hot springs, or saunas can be used for cleaning body toxins, strengthening immune responses, promoting deep relaxation, and calming the mind. Any detoxification program using natural sweats should start with at least one sweat weekly; increase the frequency to your own individual tolerance level.

In many healing traditions, the process of mobilizing the self to deal with poisoning is regarded as linked to the spiritual dimension. Sincere questions may be asked about the meaning embedded in receiving this affliction, and various rituals of purification (like prayers or sweats) may be engaged. Assistance may be requested from the dream self, or an external spiritual advisor, to determine the nature of the poisoning and the best possible course for healing.

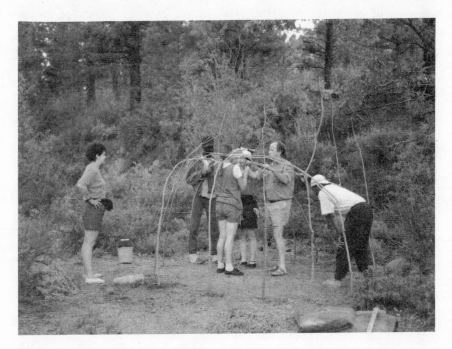

Building a sweat lodge. (photo: Tsolo)

7

Managing
Out-of-Control Experiences

Cultivating balance can be a starting point on the road back to firm ground and gaining a measure of control.

In this chapter I will talk about applying the strategy of cultivating balance in some aspects of living where imbalance may be most severe. Post-traumatic stress imbalances of this nature include nightmares, rage episodes, intrusive recall experiences, and despair. In my work I have found these to be the types of imbalances that cause the most serious difficulties for those who experience them. The common thread linking these experiences is the subjective feeling that there is "nothing you can do" when they occur, that they are completely out of your control.

The strategy of cultivating balance can be used as a starting point on the road back to firm ground and gaining a measure of control. We will be looking at three kinds of out-of-control experiences in the following sections from a position that does not see them as cancerous growths upon the personality that need to be surgically removed or irradiated away. Instead, we will view them from a position where they appear as expressions of imbalance caused by inner war. In using this strategy you will be asking yourself questions about the sort of battles you might be fighting inside yourself, and considering the options you might have available in negotiating greater peace and balance.

Traumatic Nightmares and Balance

Dreams are a creative product of human consciousness, and many individuals who have not lived through overwhelming events have experienced nightmares that elicit fear-reactions. Traumatic nightmares, however, have a special quality. For one thing, unresolved or unintegrated traumatic events (which includes events that cannot be remembered, and events that have not in other ways been accepted as something that the self lived through) may produce nightmares that are repeated frequently over many years. For another, traumatic nightmares tend to replay or reenact a traumatic event, almost as if watching a recording of the real-life prior event, with much less creative editing or use of symbolic images than in other nightmares not of this type. Such frequently repeated, anxiety producing dreams, as well as clusters of dreams with a similar stressful message, can be very debilitating. If you frequently experience dreams with a high fear/violence/anxiety content that replays elements of a traumatic event, your ability to have a relaxing and refreshing sleep may be greatly reduced. **Insufficient or poor quality sleep can cause severe imbalance through mental and physical exhaustion, producing such visible symptoms as increased irritability, general fatigue, inability to concentrate, memory lapses, and significant depression.**

In the short-term, movement towards balance includes finding a way to get sufficient sleep. If you do not find a way to sleep, other goals in your life will be more difficult to achieve. Although prescription sleep medication is not a way to find out why it is difficult for you to sleep, it can be very useful in providing short-term relief while you are tackling this question. Sedative herbal teas may also prove useful for those who do not choose to take prescription drugs. Alcohol and various controlled substances have also been widely used for this purpose, but this is very dangerous because using substances in this way is likely to reinforce long-term addiction behaviors. Tricyclic antidepressant medication (prescription only) has also proven useful for some trauma survivors with sleep disturbance in helping procure a sustained sleep. Sweating through sauna or soaking in hot water before bedtime is also widely reported as useful. Bath additives such as epsom salts or herbal plants (catnip-Nepeta cataria, peppermint-Mentha piperita, comfrey-Symphytum officinale, to name just a few plants I enjoy) are also worth experiencing to test if they are helpful for you. To use these herbs, take two large handfuls of herb materials, place in two to four quarts of boiling water, remove from heat, steep five minutes, strain, and add liquid to bath water.

For those who choose to use no ingested substances, hard physical exercise, self-hypnosis, fresh air, and tranquil natural environments have also been reported as helpful for some individuals. If you cannot sleep, choose to find some method to enhance your sleep as a high priority. **Sleeping is as essential to maintaining your natural balance as eating, drinking, and breathing.**

Beyond the need for sleep, there is the question as to why recurring nightmares are happening in your life now. Repeated nightmares have some special meaning. The most basic meaning is that they are somehow important to you, the person who is producing them in your mind. When you are spending much of your sleep time focused on particular dream images, then in some way you are sending a message to yourself. The message is to pay attention to the particular meanings that are associated with these images in your dreams. If your dreams are filled with war and you awaken feeling as though you have fought a battle, then the mind that produced those dreams is in some way requesting that you pay attention to the war that is still raging inside.

Such dreams are both the record of the war experiences you have known and reminders that in cultivating balance now you are the only person in position to negotiate peace. Using the hidden meanings in your dreams as signposts pointing towards your healing pathway can be a very difficult and slow process, because such exploration may lead back through the most painful and frightening experiences you have known.

Working with Fear-Dreams

It is hard to choose to pay attention to the most uncomfortable things in our lives, and most of us choose not to do so. When our dreams feel out-of-control, however, as in nightmares, it seems as if we have no choice: they appear to be forcing us to pay attention at some level to our inner war. Usually we stop paying attention as soon as we wake up from a nightmare: we push our thoughts in another direction as quickly and fully as possible.

Applying the practice of cultivating balance to the work of dealing with nightmares requires a process including several elements:

1. Become conscious (aware in your waking thoughts) of what is happening in your nightmares.
2. Ask yourself about what it would take to negotiate peace concerning the inner battle that your dream is requesting you pay attention to.
3. Discover ways to apply the answers you find to how you live now.

In practical experience, carrying out this unfolding process takes place over months or years. There are no sure-fire shortcuts or pain-free methods: this is hard work. It is appropriate to compare it to choosing to go to a dentist for a difficult root canal operation: doing the work is uncomfortable, but neglecting it can produce even greater discomfort.

One reason this work is difficult has to do with the nature of the "unusual experiences" that may be revealed in your dreams. If these experiences occurred in a combat zone, you may not have had sufficient opportunity to proceed through the various stages of emotional reaction that normally occur for human beings when something overwhelming has happened: denial (I don't believe it happened), anger (I'm really pissed off that it happened), and grief (I'm really hurt that it happened). These feelings may need to be felt and acknowledged before it becomes possible to reach a more balanced stage that has been called "acceptance" (I can accept what happened in a way that lets me turn my attention to the rest of my life), or an "attitude of allowing" (I can allow how it is to be as it is).

If your dreams bring back things that have happened that were overwhelming, you may need to "work through" your feelings of denial, anger, and grief before you can accept what happened then in a balanced way. This type of "working through" can leave you very vulnerable and stimulate feelings of guilt, shame, rage, and depression along the way.

It is for this reason that many trauma survivors who have done this type of self-exploration caution others that "it can get worse before it gets better." In simple terms this means that to regain the best in your life it may be necessary to spend some time coming to peace with the worst that is present. It is very helpful to have access to a safe and quiet place, people who care, and someone who understands this type of work while you are doing it. Working with a therapist, joining a group of peers exploring their dreams, and notifying your loved ones about what you are doing are all good ideas that can help make your "root canal"-type exploration provide the most favorable outcome as quickly as possible. These are some action-oriented strategies that could be called useful Western approaches to moving this process along. Eastern approaches that teach stillness or moving meditation forms can also be useful vehicles for locating your resistances to inner peace.

How do you learn what is happening in your dreams? The easiest way, of course, is to simply remember them as you wake up. Since many individuals do not naturally remember their dreams, it is worth describing other clues that may indicate the presence of combat nightmares. If you wake up sweating and anxious, then in the absence of other causes (such as a physical illness or sleeping in an overheated room) it is likely you have been dreaming about something stress-producing. If you have a bed-partner, the person may be able to tell you something about how your body behaves while you are dreaming.

If you are forcefully moving your body while asleep, this is a likely indication of anxiety in your dream sequence. Any words you speak while having such dreams are also clues about the kind of experience you were paying attention to. If you were speaking words that are linked to your combat experiences, then that is what you were paying attention to while you were dreaming.

If you are having these kinds of dream-reactions and cannot remember your dreams, you may choose to do some work to become more aware of your dream content. It is a commonly held belief among people who do not remember dreams that they do not have dreams; however, the evidence clearly indicates that all human beings dream during extended sleep. Some of us are better skilled than others at linking our waking and dreaming experiences.

If you choose to work on remembering your dreams, there are a number of activities you can begin:

a. Start a dream journal.

Keep a pencil and paper close by your bed, as well as a dim light that is easily switched on. Train yourself to write down what happened in your dream as soon as you wake up. You can use a tape recorder instead if that is easier for you. You can increase your dream awareness by choosing to make a record while your recollections are most sharp.

If you cannot recall any dream or dream fragments, you might try to wake yourself up during your dreams with the aid of an alarm clock or a friend. If you frequently awaken between midnight and 2 a.m., for example, you can experiment by setting your alarm variously at midnight, twelve thirty, and one a.m. If you can wake yourself up while you are engaged in a dream sequence, it may be easier to recall details of what was happening in the dream.

If you have a bed-partner who can recognize when you are dreaming by your movements, this person can wake you up during your dream sequence. Since at these times your reflexes may be highly activated by the stressful dream, anyone who is going to wake you up should take care to protect themselves from any defensive motions that you might make as you are awakening. A verbal request to wake up is best. If it is necessary to use physical contact to wake you, this should be done gently by using steadily increasing firm pressure to a foot. The person waking you up should take care to avoid positioning their body where it could be hurt by any sudden motion you might make, and should identify themselves as they are awakening you. Rough jerking, shaking, or jabbing motions should be avoided. When you wake up, immediately write down your recollections. You can also use the writing exercise described in Chapter 8 to search for important dream events that have happened in your life.

b. Focus the mind.

Professionals trained in the use of hypnosis and other mind-focusing methods can instruct you in ways to remember your dreams. You can also study any of the various methods of self-hypnosis in service of this goal. Meditation is also recommended as a way to enhance dream clarity and recall. There are now several books available that are filled with useful information about working directly with your own dreams.

c. Join a dream group.

Frequently it is easier to develop this skill when participating in a like-minded group. You can search for a group of individuals with similar interest by inquiring of professionals in your area, or you could start a leaderless group. **Dream groups can be very helpful as a support system while you are learning to "work through" the inner battles that are displayed in your dreams.**

Once you have a reasonably accurate record of what is occurring within your dreams (the action while the dream is going on), you can begin to ask yourself questions about why you are paying so much attention to this particular action. If the dream content is filled with the most overwhelming events that have happened in your life, then this may be the last thing in the world you would choose to think about when you are awake. However, if you wish to learn what your dreams are telling you, you must face this line of questioning eventually. You do not need to push yourself. At your own pace and when you are ready, you can turn your attention toward solving the puzzle about what you might be telling yourself. If in your dream you find yourself hating someone or something, where is that hatred coming from? If you find someone else in a rage at you, what caused this rage? If there are persons present in your dream that you once knew but are now gone, what are they asking or demanding of you and why? If you feel fear, then fear of what? Why do you fear that thing?

When you choose to cast your questions into the pool of your dream self, the answers can begin to emerge. Remember: the point of all this inquiry is to learn more about how your individual "life tree," with its particular environmental circumstances, can best reach with root and branches toward the nourishment you need. Dreamwork is one valid approach pathway, and expert help makes it easier. In learning from dreams, it is useful to be able to talk with others. If you become too involved with these powerful happenings in your inner world, it can be difficult to function in the outer world. Although there are multiple cases of spontaneous insight derived from dreams throughout history, dream-work remains an area where it is much easier to generate insight when working with others than alone. This is partly because of the overwhelming nature of the unusual experiences such dreams contain, and partly because you can refine and test your ideas about dream-meanings by sharing them with others on a similar journey and with any other people you trust.

If in doing your dream-work you remember information about previous stressful experiences that you have not been able to recall clearly, you may reexperience strong feelings, such as guilt, anger, fear or horror, that you felt during that experience. It is also possible to react strongly to memories of experiences during which you felt numb. These strong feelings are a major reason most people are unwilling to examine dream content thoroughly. It is also why it is very important to have learned some helpful rebalancing methods to use as needed while doing this work.

Whatever it is that you have paid attention to in your dreams, one way to transform the impact of negative feelings about what happened before is to extract some meaning that can be applied now.

This type of dreamwork has been documented as a creative wellspring of inspiration for artists, philosophers, healers, inventors, and just plain folks throughout recorded history. It can also be used to influence and modulate one's reactions to recurring traumatic nightmares.

Dreamwork: A Case Study

I will give a real-life example to illustrate how this can work. Before I do that, I would like to describe how I came to choose this example to write about, because I believe it is a very serious decision to report about the deep wound of another person in this way. When I first wrote about this subject, I constructed a hypothetical example to describe how to do this type of dreamwork. I did this because I did not have permission from anyone who had shared their story with me to write about it, and also because I was not sure if writing about someone else's nightmare would be as beneficial for the dreamer as it would be in increasing the clarity of my book.

That has changed now. One who shared his story with me has given such permission, and I have watched this person gain something very substantial from telling about his dream-work and his life to others. In his case I no longer have uncertainty that writing his story will cause him distress. As he stated, "If you can say anything that's going to make it easier for anybody else who has experienced these kinds of things, do it and that's fine with me." I offer this lengthy explanation because if I am going to model the behavior of choosing to write about someone else's story, I must also inform my readers that such choices should be made with utmost care, sensitivity, and "checking in" with the needs of the story-owner. Our society does not have a very good track record in offering this level of respect to trauma survivors. Developing this respect is essential if we are to create "safe" environments where survivors feel comfortable enough in speaking about their successes to choose to teach the rest of us how to do it.

Now for our example: M is a Korean war veteran. He served as a combat medic with several MASH units and was involved in some of the most violent and casualty-filled battles of that war. He was exposed to many overwhelming events.

One particular event had made a very deep impression on him. This event had replayed as a traumatic nightmare with some degree of regularity for approximately 35 years at the time we met. M reported that there were times when the dream replayed every night for weeks at a stretch, and other times when the dream was absent for months. He invariably woke up from this dream with a severe anxiety reaction, sometimes night sweats, inability to return to sleep, and compulsive scratching behavior. He reported feeling severe depression, guilt, and uncertainty as to whether his life was worth living.

The first time I met M he had experienced this dream recently. He was brought to see me by a friend who was concerned by the intensity of his anxiety reaction. He was not very coherent at that time, and it took several subsequent talks to understand the elements of this traumatic nightmare.

In the dream, M returned to a particular wartime event. He was stationed at the time with an emergency medical unit at a South Korean warzone military airfield. This airfield serviced aircraft from many nations of the international coalition fighting against the Communists. M's dream recalled a particular daytime event while he was on duty at that airfield. A South African pilot (South Africa, M explained to me, had fought as our ally in the Korean War) had just filled his tanks and taken off from the airfield. Something went wrong just after takeoff, and the plane crashed on the airfield grounds. M raced in a jeep with a medical team to the crash site, where the plane had already exploded. As they arrived, M could hear the screaming of the pilot, who was trapped in the airplane cockpit and could not get out. M tried to approach the aircraft but could not because of the intense heat. He heard screams of agony from the trapped pilot, and he knew this pilot's life could not be saved. He stood on the hood of the medical jeep, pulled his sidearm from the holster he wore, and emptied it at the pilot in order to end his life and pain more quickly. He remembered the pilot looking at him as this happened.

This overwhelming event had replayed many hundreds of times in M's nightmares. He reported very little variation in his experience of this dream; it was as if a movie of this time had been taken and replayed in his dream life. The dream almost always ended with M's action, and a sense that the pilot's eyes were looking at him. He reported that his reaction upon awakening was severely unbalancing.

M's work with this dream proceeded slowly. As a few weeks passed, he gradually was able to describe his dreams to me and to the friend who had brought him. As more time went by, he began to share this with other combat veterans in the traumatic nightmare dream group that he had joined. It became clear to him that he was carrying a large load of guilt about his participation in this event, and it also became clear to him — through the feedback he received from other dream group members — that this was clearly a situation where he was experiencing "a sane reaction to living through an insane situation." It was great relief for M to sit with a group of listeners who did not believe he was crazy because he had this recurring dream. After 35 years of doing his best to hide this dream and being judged harshly where he could not, this peer support was a new experience. Although it did not seem to affect the nightmare or his immediate post-nightmare reactions at this point, the knowledge that there was support in the world for his difficult internal experience made a significant difference in his depression and self-esteem. As he was doing this inner work, M began to volunteer to help as he could with the difficulties of others in the groups he was participating in. His ability to return to balance following anxiety reactions gradually improved, although he still had a tendency to dissociate back to the Korean warzone if too much emphasis and attention was placed on his experiences.

After several months M appeared ready to do further work on this nightmare. He asked if there was anything he could do to affect this recurring nightmare. I told him I didn't know, and we could try. We did some individual work exploring his relationship with the South African pilot, and what most bothered him in the dream sequence. It turned out that what bothered him the most was the image of the pilot's eyes looking at him, just before his life had ended. M felt there was an accusation in that look that had haunted him for many years. We began to question what might be needed for M to feel comfortable that he had an appropriate response to that accusation. He knew logically, he said, that the man's life could not have been saved, and that he was in mortal agony. Emotionally, though, he could not answer that accusatory look and had hidden from it.

I began to ask M to question what there could be that might move this relationship in the direction of peaceful rest. M began to express his deep feelings about the event: his anger in finding himself in such a powerless position to save the pilot's life, the connection of this powerlessness to other such experiences in M's life, his compassion for the pilot's suffering, as well as the suffering of all the wounded soldiers he had encountered; his fear that the South African pilot was angry at him for not doing more to save him. Eventually we brought M's attention back to that very difficult choice-moment when he had to decide whether to act passively and listen to the pilot burn slowly, or act forcefully, as he actually did. I tried to help him see this event from the position of an observer, rather than from his position within in the event, so as to lessen the retraumatization caused by placing attention on that event.

M realized that in that situation he had had no good choices. This realization was very important for him, because until that time he had always suspected that somehow he should have done better, that the situation was somehow his fault. In realizing that he had truly lived through an experience where there were no good choices available to him, he could see more clearly why he had made the choice he made. He had chosen the most compassionate choice available, by his standard, and the choice in line with his duty to relieve suffering. He realized that if he faced the same awful situation again, he could find no better choice than the one he had made. He had not known or been able to see any of this at the time, however, and what he had done to live with his memory had been to numb his compassionate heart in a way that held long-lasting effects.

In sensing all this from a different vantage point, M was ready to encounter the image of the pilot's eyes in a new way. He felt he didn't have to be so afraid of the pilot now: he had done the best he could by him. He was now willing to explore this further, with me in the role of the pilot, to get practice discovering what he had to say to this man whose image he had carried with him for so long.

M needed to express his sorrow, it turned out, that the whole situation had happened at all; he also needed to tell this other man that he had done what he did to help him and not to hurt him. He was sorry, he said, if the pilot was angry with him for what he had done — he had been angry with himself, too, he told the pilot-memory, and was just now realizing he had done the best he could to help the pilot. M found a way to state all this clearly in our imagination exercises. I asked him to remember what he had said and to say it again when he next found himself in that familiar dream-encounter. I suggested that he might even ask for this dream to come, just before he went to bed, but this was too much for a man who had been avoiding this experience so long. M said he didn't want to ask for this dream to come, but he would try to remember what to do when it did come.

And that is what happened. The next night, the nightmare replayed, and M was caught in its grip as usual. Near the end, though, when looking at the pilot's eyes, he suddenly remembered enough of his dreamwork so that he found his voice. In the dream, while looking at the pilot, he said the things he had to say. And, to his surprise, the pilots" eyes — which had invariably appeared to pierce him with anger and accusation — appeared to smile at him. M woke up from this recurring dream energized and without his usual anxiety reaction. He knew something important had happened.

M continued to work with this dream and, over time, it lost its ability to elicit a fear-reaction in him. The sequence still replays, from time to time, but no longer holds the "haunting" and fear-arousing quality it once did. M knows that the pilot knows they are allies, and the confusion between them has been laid to rest. The dream lost the ability to throw M off-balance.

It is now 6 years since this dreamwork was initiated, and the results reported have remained stable. The deep healing with this dream affected other aspects of M's life as well. I will relate his words, as he spoke them to others when he shared this dream publicly: "After this happened, I shut down and lost the ability to love. I made a lot of mistakes and hurt many people, especially my family and friends. I didn't know why. After doing this work on the dream, and other places I was afraid, I really learned how to love again, and that's been the difference between feeling dead and feeling alive."

Dissociation, "Flashbacks" and Balance

When dissociative experiences happen in your life, there is a serious loss of balance. Something has affected the boundaries of yourself in a way that has changed your perceptions of what is "self" and what is "not-self." **In the case of traumatic flashback-type dissociation, something that happened before is capturing your attention in a way that is more real and more alive for you than what is happening now.** When your attention is focused in this way, you make choices about what you will do that would have been acceptable choices back in the situation that happened before but very poor choices for dealing with what is really happening now. Using "combat-mode" aggression and experiencing self as living in an active combat zone is an often reported combat-type dissociative state; using a passive and hyper-erotic coping style and experiencing self as living in an active sexual abuse event is an often reported sexual abuse-type dissociative state.

There are several keys to learning how to minimize the frequency and impact of dissociative experiences in your life. Although many trauma victims have reported that such experiences seem to simply happen without any identifiable cause, reports from those trauma survivors who have worked to regain balance during such experiences consistently agree that there are telltale "clues" that show up before this type of experience occurs. These clues are the types of messages that I have been discussing as the signs of loss of balance: tight muscles, anxious thoughts, particular body sensations associated with traumatic events, intense emotions, and in some cases activation of the "fight or flight" command.

In other words, stress has usually been building for some time before you reach the point where a flashback is produced. **Prolonged general stress can weaken you and leave you more vulnerable to reacting intensely to stressful events.**

Flashbacks are often stimulated by "triggering events." A triggering event is something that happens in the present moment — often unexpectedly — that in some way reminds you of what happened then. For example, under certain conditions, noises, smells, sights, thoughts, or feelings that are associated with what happened before can act as triggers to flashbacks. Triggering events are not only connected to what is happening in your psychological environment. For those heavily exposed to toxic chemicals and currently experiencing chemical sensitivity disorder, exposure to toxic substances in the air, water, and food supply may stress the body severely enough to act as a triggering event. Triggering events will be able to knock you off-balance more easily where you are already weakened by stress. This is another reason why cultivating balance is so important.

If you are having flashbacks, this means that you are sometimes having trouble in accurately perceiving what is happening now; some unusual experience you have lived through is exerting such a strong "gravitational pull" on your attention that you lose the ability to pay attention to what is happening now. Flashbacks are in fact a serious sign of imbalance, a signal that there is some important work to be done in learning to plant your feet more firmly in the here-and-now. Remember it is your mind that is producing this warning sign; it is a clue from inside yourself that this is really important in some way. The clue is somehow pointing to an area of experience where you have not developed an "attitude of allowing" concerning what really happened.

Most individuals need some help to learn the skills necessary to manage these out-of-control experiences. The preventive skills that can help you deal with disassociative "flashback" experiences are gained by:

1. Learning to recognize when stress is building up inside.

2. Learning methods to reduce stress.

3. Learning to take a "timeout" and practice stress-reducing activities when you need them.

4. Learning to find ways to remind yourself not to confuse what happened then with what is happening now. It is sometimes useful when stress is high and you feel your internal pressure building to say to yourself: "This isn't_____." (Fill in the blank with the traumatic event that is pressing on your attention). With practice, this can help you strengthen your ability to stay focused on what is happening now when tensions are running so high as to remind you about what was happening before.

5. Learning to make peace with the overwhelming events that are grabbing your attention now. This is the same type of work as in learning from your nightmares; the pathways to healing are basically the same.

Rage Episodes and Balance

The state of rage is a long distance away from the state of balance. As you can demonstrate to yourself by playing Push Hands, strong anger will cause you to use your force in ways that can upset your balance easily. When you are enraged, however, you are unlikely to be very reasonable about or very willing to do much in the way of cultivating balance. During the experience of rage, internal pressure has reached a critical mass and is seeking immediate release. How can you cultivate balance to manage severe anger?

There are short-term preventive steps you can use for damage

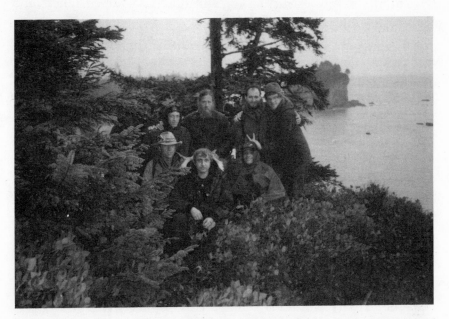

Russian and American veterans and therapists practicing balance "on the edge," coastal erratic formation, Native American tribal lands (with permission), Washington State Coast. (photo: Kostya)

control (like a fire extinguisher putting out a brush fire); also there are in-depth self-exploration methods that may lead you to the causes of your rage.

As short-term control measures, you can take preventive actions that minimize the destruction you will inflict on yourself, others, and property while enraged. These include:

a. **If you have weapons, store them with a friend or in a difficult-to-reach location.** If you are unwilling to do this, you can at least store weapon and ammunition separately. This can buy time to think about what you are doing before you are committed to any rage-driven activity. When you are enraged you may act impulsively and without thinking of consequences. A little extra pause may save you from committing actions you later regret.

   If you don't use firearms, ask yourself what type of weapons or other vessels you do use to express your anger. Do you drive an automobile at high speeds, engage in increased substance use, use your sexuality as a vehicle for aggression? In what directions can your motivation to "overcome the enemy" turn?

   Look for ways to develop preventive, "ventilating" steps you can take in the areas you turn up by the above questioning.

b. **Move yourself away from any person at whom your rage is directed.** This is called "getting some space." When you are far off your balance, it is not the best time to confront people. Even if you have legitimate anger and have been wronged, you will likely be unable to express it clearly or heal the situation while you are enraged. Such confrontations are best made when your balance is more stable. This does not mean you need to act as a meek and mild-mannered mouse; it does mean you need to gain control of your own force before you seek to use it.

c. **Find a safe place where it is okay to feel angry without needing to explain it to anyone.** This could be in a park, in your car, a room in your home, or anywhere else. Without such a place, you may find yourself releasing your rage at concerned loved ones or innocent bystanders who get in the way. Precious friends as well as total strangers can be injured by fallout from your explosions. You can minimize such injuries by releasing your anger in your safe place.

d. **Find some nondestructive activity or activities that help you "vent" or release the pressure of the anger.** Some people find strong physical activity (chopping wood, jogging, or other sweat-producing tasks) helps discharge the high internal pressure associated with rage. Others find it helpful to express their feelings to a sympathetic ear; some feel it is helpful to speak honestly to themselves by writing their feelings down while they are enraged. (They may or may not choose to show these writings to anyone else.) Taking a walk or a journey through a natural environment can also defuse the rage state and buy time to calm down.

If you already know activities like these that have worked for you, use them as needed .

If you cannot find any method to help your rage subside, you can fall back to your safe place and wait. Time and distance from nonpeaceful stimuli will be your allies in returning to balance. **Watch out for alcohol while enraged; it can fuel your rage like gasoline on a burning fire.**

If you choose in the long term to become less susceptible to periodic episodes of rage, Western healing strategies tend to suggest that you may need to develop greater insight as to the things that are happening around and inside you when anger reactions escalate. Your anger reactions may be caused by the immediate situation, by old reflexes from your "unusual experiences," or by a combination of factors. Self-exploration to find patterns where anger has shown up in your life (see Chapter 8) may help this process. Eastern healing strategies tend to suggest that gaining skill in cultivating a nonattached and peaceful state of mind can enable a person to allow strong emotions to float across the field of awareness, like a wave, without causing the person to identify with and act upon them.

If, as I suggested in Chapter 3, anger is preceded by fear, then one way to begin to question the roots of your anger is to ask yourself "What is threatening me?" when the anger reaction flares up. This type of questioning can help defuse rage that is based in projection. **Projection is a natural psychological process whereby we disown or dis-identify with some aspect of ourselves we don't like by "projecting" that aspect outside ourselves onto some other person or thing.** For example, imagine a person who is badly wounded and hurting and cannot acknowledge that situation. This person will be using a great deal of energy to hold those feelings inside, even though they may not be consciously aware of this. Suppose that another person comes along (let's call this other person "the messenger") and takes some action that somehow directs the first person's attention to the pain they are carrying. All too frequently, the reaction of the hurting person would be to project their feeling onto the messenger; that is, to perceive that the messenger is somehow responsible for the pain they are feeling. In this situation, the messenger is perceived as a real threat, "the enemy," and — if the projection is not reclaimed (which means in this example that the hurting person comes to a realization that they themselves are responsible for the pain they are feeling) — then much energy may be expended in blaming or otherwise attacking the messenger with rage-driven activity. Individuals who have great difficulty in experiencing and claiming responsibility for their feelings are at high risk of projecting onto "messengers" as a justification for expressing rage. This can be used as a less-than-desirable coping style for discharging emotions where a person has not yet learned other methods for experiencing and processing their feelings. Whether you use Eastern or Western methods to recognize the qualities of events and situations that seem to be threatening you, you can increase your ability to slow down your "fight or flight" command as you are preparing to respond to threat.

Remember that rage episodes are not events that "happen out of nowhere"; they are methods you have learned for coping with overwhelming pressures. As you extend your self-examination and more options become visible, the methods you use to cope with such unusual and overwhelming pressures can change.

8

Long-Range Reconnaissance Patrol

Searching Inside Yourself

How can you find your place in this crazy world? How can you find peace in your life? These questions may be more relevant to healing than paying attention to what's wrong with you or with the world.

In this chapter, the goal is to learn more about the story you tell yourself about who you are. In learning to fill in this story, you are learning to pay attention to more of the parts of yourself. When beginning to locate some clues about your personal path towards healing, it is not so important that you reach towards anyone else's standard of healing. Your own standards are what count here. This long range reconnaissance patrol inside yourself is designed to help you learn more about just what your own standards really are.

The task here is to take an assessment of what your life is about (I'll share a method to do this in a while). You will be looking at aspects of yourself that may be out-of-balance (such as the post-traumatic stress symptoms I have described) and aspects that are well-balanced. You will be looking for information that can help you develop "anchors" to help you weather the stormy moments in your life: the life that has brought you through your individual unusual experiences. You will be reconnoitering for the available choices that can bring acceptance and peace more powerfully into your life. To find the choices that can realistically fit, you need to search inside yourself. That is where they live.

In seeking answers that fit, it is urgent to be asking questions that have meaning for you. How can you find your place in this crazy world? How can you obtain a measure of peace in your life? Is it possible to make sense out of the ugly things that have happened? This type of questioning may be more relevant to healing than paying attention to what's wrong with you or with the world.

Balance and Self-Identity

In my work I have observed that many survivors who felt an uncomfortably limited sense of control over their lives began to develop a greater sense of control as they spent time asking themselves these questions. The purpose in asking them is to relearn the skill of speaking honestly with yourself. **You certainly cannot control everything in your life, and the place you can exert the greatest influence is within your own self:** you can control what you pay attention to inside and the choices you make there. You may have been or still may be "stuck" in certain ways of acting, thinking, or feeling. Possibly you are telling yourself that these ways of behaving are who you are. There is a strange thing about self-identity, though, about who we are: **there is more to us, than who we tell ourselves we are.** When you participate in this inquiry into self-identity, you can test this statement for yourself.

Usually we tell ourselves just parts of the story. For example, if you have a job you do well and enjoy, you may identify yourself as the successful person who does that job. If you do not have a job, you may identify yourself as unemployed and tell yourself that an "unemployed person" is who you are. You might see yourself as the parent of your children and identify yourself as family-oriented. You might identify with your home or your homelessness. Or, you might identify with a traumatic event or time period in your history and tell yourself, "I am the one who lived through that." Whatever combination of these or other things you might tell yourself, you also very likely have more parts than that. The ones you pay attention to may be real, but they are rarely the whole story. The purpose here is to reconnoiter the path of your life — the experiences you have lived through — to take a look at the happenings that helped form you into the person that lives here-and-now and to see if perhaps you can relocate some parts of yourself that you may have lost touch with over time. Some are parts that will be painful to remember; these are the places where you lost your balance, where you were knocked down somehow by life. Other parts will be very nourishing to recall; these are likely the places where you learned some of what you know about holding your balance.

Searching Inside Yourself: Strategy for Telling Your Story

It's important to begin with the basic rule that this reconnaissance is something you do for yourself and no one else. As you proceed you will need to write down your recollections, which means you will create a written record. Make sure that you keep this record safe — it is just for you. Things may come up as you proceed through this work that you wish to share with others, and that's fine. But no one else has the right to demand access to it; it's also fine if you chose not to share it with anyone. The reason for this rule is that you will be most successful in this reconnaissance when you can be most honest, and you will likely be more honest with yourself than anyone else.

In order to do this type of search, you'll need to be as accurate as you can about what you find. Your mission will be to pay attention to the terrain and report what you see. Only in this case, the terrain is your life and the only one you will report to is yourself. To begin, you will be looking through what has happened in your life, using a particular method I will explain shortly, searching for the important experiences that have happened. You will be scanning the terrain for evidence of the different kinds of experiences you have been through.

The reason for doing this is to help fill in missing pieces in the story of who you are. We all get caught up in daily routines (habits of acting, thinking, and feeling), and we identify with them. We think these ways are all there is to us, that they are the stuff that the most essential "me" is made of. "Me" is bigger than that.

The things that have happened that occupy your thoughts most often are not the whole story. If you are old enough to read this book, you've been alive a long time and have been through many experiences of different varieties. You have not only lived through some traumatic event(s), you've also been through a lot of other experiences as well. **In paying attention to what you have known, you can become more clear about what you need to know.** Many survivors have stated that in the here-and-now of their lives they do not know how to relax or to reach a place of peace. And, because repeated exposure to this way of experiencing leads such individuals to tell themselves the story: "that is who I am," you may tell yourself you cannot experience these things, that the experience of peace is not included in "who I am."

What I am going to request that you do here is to take a time out from holding so tightly to the story you have been telling yourself; time out to make sure you've got the whole story about who you are; time out to go through your life with an open mind; time out to explore. The chances are that somewhere in your life you have been happy (if only for a short while). Somewhere in your life you've felt confident and proud of who you are. There was a tendril of strength. Somewhere in your life you've felt some kind of fear and found a way beyond it. There was a victory. Somewhere in your life you have played and been relaxed. Somewhere you have tasted a good taste and found a drink that quenched your thirst. It will be helpful to find where these places are. Not so you can share them with anybody else or so anyone else can judge you, but because it is helpful for you to remember that you already know that there is more to you than the story you've let yourself see. The experiences you have had point to the skills that you have used, skills that you may not yet recognize as something useful for your life now. **It's easier to relearn something you once knew, than to learn something that you have never done before.**

One purpose of this exploration is to reclaim some of the territory of yourself that you may not be using now — to remember that it is also part of your identity — so that when you consider this idea of "me," you can tell yourself a bigger story than you were remembering before. Although I won't ask you to accept this just because I say so, I will tell you what I have observed again and again: as the story you tell yourself about who you are gets more and more filled in, you become able to make more choices about how you want to live now. Your job at this point is neither to accept or reject this statement, only to try it and see for yourself if it is helpful.

Searching Inside Yourself: A Basic Method

The writing method I will now describe can help you to regain pieces of your story. It is not a game; it is a serious psychological tool of considerable power. You are not ready to use it unless you are willing to listen to what you have to say.

In working with this kind of technique, you will have to use your imagination. You don't have to have a particularly good imagination: you just need at the minimum to know what a road looks like. Do you know what a road looks like? As long as you've got that one figured out, you can start using this method.

The first step is to imagine your life — made up of all your experiences — as if it were a road. First, you're born; that's the beginning of the road for you, here on planet Earth. Each place you've been and event you've known exists along the road you have travelled. There's more of the road, untravelled as yet, but we will not look that way now. You were born, and the road started there. It stretches to now. Your reconnaissance assignments will be along this stretch of the road.

You're going to look at some of the things that have happened along the road. It would be best if you got a paper and pencil ready at this point, because you will be writing down some information about what you observe along the road. You won't want to write down too much. When you observe some important scenery along the road, you'll want to write down just enough so that you'll have a record of it. Here's how it works:

> First, imagine yourself sitting up in the distant hills, over-looking the road. The road of your life. You will not be on the road; you are removed from it, looking down at this road from higher ground. You will be looking along the road, checking the scenery, looking at the things that have happened in your life. At first, you will look for the things that really made a difference in shaping you as you are.

Before you begin, I will explain how you write down your observations on this reconnaissance.

> Imagine, for example, that you suffered a serious loss when you were 6 years old — such as a loss of a family member. This might well be an important event in your life, something that made a difference. When you scan along your road, it might be a piece of the scenery that you would notice. Another possibility might be that when you were 6 years old, you met another child who became your friend and taught you important things. This could per-haps also be something that made a difference in your life.

When it is your life, it is for you to decide. These important events can happen at any age in your life. You do not need to follow

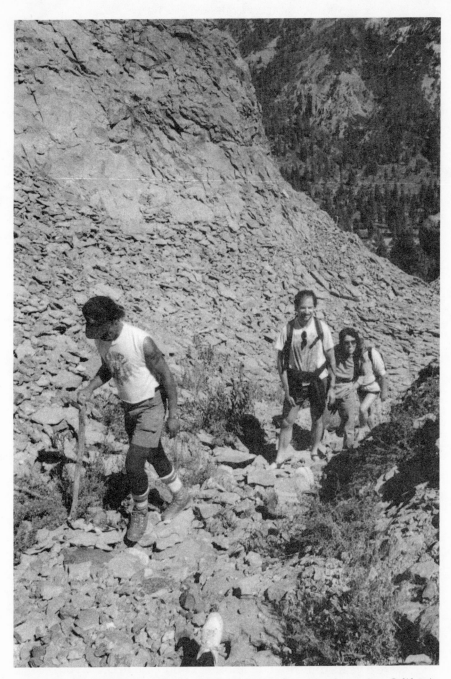

Ascending devastation zone to high ground, wilderness demonstration project, California Sierras. (photo: Tsolo)

any particular formula. You are requested here to give your mind free rein, to follow the scenery along the road, looking for the things that made a difference. As you tell yourself about your own story and reencounter some of your important scenery, you make a record of what you observe. You just need to write enough so that the key word or words that you write will remind you of the scenery you are seeing on that piece of the road.

Going back to the examples, the road watcher who lost some family when he was six might simply write "family"; he knows what experience that refers to. The one who made an important friend when he was six might write "friend" or the friend's name. **Write just enough so you'll know what you're talking about when you refer back to it later.** Since you're not writing this for anyone else, there is no need to be detailed.

Here's how to use this method. In your mind's eye, imagine a picture of the road. You are not on the road; you are up in the hills or other high ground, and the road appears in the distance. The road starts where you were born and stretches through all the territory up until now. You are not on any part of the road; you are reconnoitering it from a distance. You may see a flat and straight road, or it may be very curvy. It may have peaks, valleys, or just about anything.

To start your reconnaissance, you will lift your imaginary binoculars to the start of the road from your vantage point on high ground. At the same time, you say to yourself, "I was born there." Then begin to sweep along the road with your binoculars as you say to yourself, "and after that. . . ." Look for whatever shows up along the road of your life that made a difference. Do not attempt to structure your thoughts; just look at what comes up. Do not force your thoughts, worrying, "I should probably include this or that." Just imagine yourself scanning along the road while you hold this thought about the important things that made a difference in shaping you as you are and see what shows up in your field of view.

Repeat this procedure along your entire road up to now. Try to limit yourself to ten key items or so on this first reconnaissance. This will help you focus on some really important events. Take 20 or 30 minutes and see what you come up with. One of the curious things about this reconnaissance is that even though you are looking in just one direction along the road — from the past towards the present — you do not always remember the things that made a difference in the order they happened. When you have read these instructions to this point, you have the information necessary to take your first scan. When you are ready, give it a try.

When you have finished, look now at your key words: Do you identify some with positive feelings and beautiful scenery along your road? Do you identify some with negative feelings and ugly scenery along your road? Which ones recall experiences where you felt good about who you are? Which recall experiences where you felt the opposite?

The answers to these questions contain clues about what these experiences mean to you inside. As you have recorded these experiences, you see, you have been reclaiming parts of you, experiences that you are intimately familiar with because you were there. So as you look back and remember the friend that made a difference, or enemy, or loved one, or idea — or whatever else you came up with — you can ask yourself: "Do I want more of that in my life now? Do I want less?"

You might see if the keywords you have identified form a mixture of experiences that you would judge from your present vantage point as "good" and "bad," "positive" and "negative," "beautiful" and "ugly." If they appear heavily weighted in one direction, you have gained information that the story you are telling yourself about your life is focused in that direction. This means it is possible that your individual "life tree," in adapting to your life circumstances, may have once needed to reach away from certain aspects of your story, aspects you may now be ready to reclaim. This type of scanning can give you clues about where you are paying attention and where you are not.

Your answers are a beginning. They are a way to start telling yourself what you are looking for and what you do not want to look at. If you have spent a great deal of your time with your attention focused on scenery that you don't want to look at, it is easy to feel like you have no control. As you begin to get some information and some insight about the kind of experiences you want more of now, you will be better able to steer your life in the direction of the things you need to maintain balance. As you do that, you gain more control.

Unfinished Business

As you make your scans and find events that made a difference, you may notice that some of them have a particular quality associated with them that can be termed "unfinished business." Events that are related to "unfinished business" can stimulate some inner reaction that is unbalancing when you turn your attention their way. You may have listed many events that had a major impact on your life. If, when you remember them, it is easy to look, observe, and put those memories "back on the shelf" in your mind, chances are good that those events do not contain "unfinished business," and that you have made peace with whatever happened and have laid it to rest. Events related to "unfinished business," though, tend to evoke some kind of reaction: anger, fear, love, sadness, or some other feeling. Places where you locate this "unfinished business" can be very important clues as to where to direct your future peace-making activities.

Searching for Inner Peace

Next is an exercise of a different type. The basic idea is the same: you will again imagine yourself on high ground, looking at the road of your life, and scanning along the road. This time, instead of looking for everything that happened that made a difference, you will be looking for a specific type of scenery that made a difference.

During this next reconnaissance, I'd like you to scan for the places in your life where you have felt natural and at peace — places you were doing what you felt you were supposed to be doing, where your balance felt most firm and made a difference in who you are. You will be looking for those expereiences that held some quality of nourishment, connectedness, sacredness as you lived them.

Perhaps, for example, you may observe yourself at three years of age playing with your favorite toy. If it truly made a difference, write it down. Nothing should be judged as too silly, too trivial, or too anything else. You alone will use this record; if you are engaged on this mission then you have chosen to learn just what kind of story you are telling yourself about you. Any experiences that pop up, while you are scanning along the road are part of the story. So if you find your scan hovering on an idyllic fishing vacation, a positive sexual experience, a good idea, work on some project, a flower in your garden, whatever — write it down. Again, take 20-30 minutes and try to limit yourself to items of particular strength.

When you have completed this exercise, you will remember that there have been moments in your life — even if they were a long time ago — when you felt good. If you came up with a blank sheet (i.e. nothing has ever felt good), then you have gained some basic information about the story you have been telling yourself, namely, that life never feels good. In this special case, you may need to do some special work to remember the best in your life. Try this exercise again — only instead of looking for high "peaks" or wonderful moments, just look for the time where there was the most calm and the least discomfort in your life. This can be a starting point in helping you find the places in your experience where you were most comfortable with yourself. For those who are experiencing post-traumatic distress, it can be very difficult to locate the places in one's experience that held nourishment, peace, or positive spiritual resonances. One person who tried this exercise remarked to me that their road looked like a concrete airport runway and nothing else. I asked that attention be turned to looking for any places where there might be cracks in the concrete, and a blade of grass had sprung up. If one's life has been filled with "nonpeace," look for the places along the road where the "nonpeace" was a little less and made a difference.

If you did come up with some observations on this scan, take a moment to consider what is on your list. The chances are good that you would like to have these sort of experiences in your life now. Even if they happened a long time ago, you see, you are telling yourself the story of the experiences you appreciate now. So the person who is doing the appreciating, the one who has chosen these particular memories out of all that has happened, is the you that is alive in the present.

You are beginning to get some clues about the sort of experiences that might bring more meaning to your life. This does not mean that you need to try to relive the past. That is not possible. It simply means that you have located some experiences in your past that tell you what makes it feel good to be alive. As you remember those experiences, they may help you face decisions about how to live now. They give you a sort of homing beacon to take readings from when you are facing the tough choices. You can ask yourself, "If I choose to go in this direction, will it move me towards those good feelings?" I like to think of these places along our road as spiritual "anchors," places that are like safe havens within our minds. They have power to help us return to balance when we are afraid or otherwise paying attention to what is "not okay" in our experience. Using them is like a form of inner Push Hands.

Because the knowledge of your innermost needs and feelings come from inside you, and not from anyone else, they are authentic, legitimate, and to be trusted as arrows pointing the way along your healing path.

Even if you have not been able to get at this knowledge for a long time, it is still there. Focusing your attention on the scenery on your road where you experienced your own balance may make it easier to make choices that help you get back there.

If you remembered a time when you felt very relaxed, for example, and you have not been able to relax for a long time, then you can help yourself relax now by imagining that you are back in the experience where you once relaxed. This is no trick; it is a way to use the knowledge you have gained through your life. You are attempting to import something useful from prior experience into the here-and-now.

Using your imagination to relax in this way is similar to using the relaxation exercise I discussed in Chapter 4. Paying attention to relaxing thoughts sends a relaxation message to the brain, which relays this message throughout the body. If you have difficulty in holding your attention on relaxing thoughts, focusing on relaxing experiences in the past is a good way to overcome that difficulty.

Searching for Inner Wounds

For the next reconnaissance, use extra caution. Follow the same basic method as before. This time, you will be looking at some of the ugly scenery along your road, the places where painful and frightening things have happened — the places where you most seriously lost your balance.

This type of reconnaissance is the one you are most likely to avoid, because it is very uncomfortable to recognize and pay attention to our fear and our pain. There is no need to push yourself: when you are ready, you will stop avoiding this scenery. When you are not ready, it is best to be honest with yourself.

To do this reconnaissance, scan along your road and stop to write key words where you find places where pain or other ugliness happened and made a difference.

Because of the special nature of this type of scenery, you may have some strong reactions. If this occurs, make a record of what you were thinking/feeling when the reaction occurred. This is another clue about what is important to you. When you are finished with this reconnaissance, use your "internal radar" and scan your muscles for signs of tension. It is common to tense up when doing this difficult work. If you find a high tension level, take the time to breathe back to balance before you move on to something else.

If you have an extremely strong reaction as you observe this scenery along your road, break off the exercise and return to it later. Try to be honest with yourself about what you were observing on your road when the reaction happened. If this exercise is too difficult for you to complete at this time, you may consider finding some outside help in paying attention to these parts of the story. The people you trust the most and the people with similar scenery in their lives are good places to start a search for the right kind of help.

Please understand that if you have lived through "unusual experiences" that were overwhelming, it may be very difficult for you to fill in the parts of your story that can be found in this exercise. You may experience a very detailed reconnaissance, or you may feel as though you cannot see the terrain clearly. Sometimes seeing this terrain clearly takes time, like peeling an onionskin one layer at a time, little by little.

This is not an easy or comfortable job. Almost every trauma survivor I have encountered who has done this type of work agrees that "It gets harder before it gets easier."

Though we might wish it otherwise, this is an accurate statement. I know of no way to take the hurt out of that which is painful. Yet it is also true that it does get easier. Your healing pathway can lead through being stuck with uncomfortable feelings to a more balanced position. If there are hidden dark spots inside that are very painful, they may need to see the light of day in order for healing to happen.

Searching for the Open Heart

Now for another type of reconnaissance. This time, you will be looking for the scenery where love occurred inside you. It may have turned out with a happy ending, and it may have been disastrous. How it turned out is not the central question here. Look for the places along your road where love happened and made a difference. It doesn't need to be sexual love — it could also be love of a parent, a friend, an animal, an idea, a place, or generalized compassion without an object — anything that fired up your heart in a way that really counted. Repeat the basic procedure: Start on the high ground and observe your road and scan forward in time, repeating: "I was born, and after that. . . ." Sweep along the road, and find the scenery where love happened in your life and made a difference.

You may have had a terrible childhood, and perhaps you can remember no loving scenery until after you left home. Scan on. Or, you may remember love as a child, but nothing since. Keep scanning. Something happened, somewhere. Even if it is not what happened along most of your road, there are places where you can find that scenery, somewhere. Some kind of love, of caring, that made a difference. Find those experiences, and record key words. Again take 20-30 minutes, and limit yourself to the most important items.

Reclaiming Our Selves

The point of doing these exercises is to help reclaim some parts of your story that may be useful in meeting the tasks you face now. You have seen that there are many experiences that played a role in shaping you into you. Perhaps some were very ugly; perhaps some were not so ugly. You have seen that there were times when you actually felt good, and times when you experienced love. So if you have been telling yourself that you are a person who doesn't know how to feel good, or a person who cannot love or be loved, perhaps this will stretch the story you've been telling yourself a little bit, not because anyone else has told you anything but because you are learning to give yourself clues about more of the whole story. **You are a human being with the ability to live many, many different ways.**

You may also choose to use this inward scanning method to fill in other parts of your story. Choose any subject that is important to you as the "filter" you place on your scan. If you are having a problem with anger, for example, you might want to look at the scenery along your road where anger has happened and made a difference. If you are working on a relationship, you might want to recheck the relationships along your road. You might need to take a look at what has happened along your road in relation to work, or money, or your body. Your road belongs to you: you can retrieve what you need from it when you are ready.

9

Healing with Ancestors and Old Ghosts

The unconscious influence of the attitudes of our family stays with us throughout our lives. It can shape our decisions, our values, and our ability to experience peace.

Overwhelming events are not the whole story about PTS or about the influences that have helped shape your identity. As your explorations may have demonstrated, a variety of people, places, and events have made a difference in shaping your outlook and your ability to maintain balance under different conditions.

One place where most of us learned how to live was in our family of origin — from our mothers and fathers and those others who may have acted in these roles during our early life. It is quite the "usual experience" for us humans, when young and impressionable, to copy the actions, attitudes, and ways of expressing thoughts and feelings that were used by our parents. This is called "modelling" — it means we learn to model our actions upon the actions of those around us, and especially those whom we love and respect.

At a tender age, we may have sought to win parental approval by behaving and thinking in ways that pleased them, or — where we rejected their values — we may have taken great pains not to behave or think as they did. In either case, how they related to the world around them exerted a great influence upon us. Much of this influence may remain unconscious; we are not aware of it.

Ancestor Inheritance

The unconscious influence of the attitudes of our family stays with us throughout our lives. I refer to this type of family inheritance as "ancestor inheritance," since it can influence us not only directly through our mothers, fathers, and immediate family but also indirectly through the lives of our more distant forebears. It can shape our decisions, our values, and our ability to experience peace. Because of this powerful and hidden influence upon our unconscious beliefs (the things we believe in, without being aware that we believe in them), ancestor inheritance is another important area of inquiry for those of us who wish to extend our ability to maintain balance.

If you came from a family where it was considered a sign of weakness to express emotions, for example, then you may have learned to "stuff" your true feelings at an early age. If this occurred and you then experienced overwhelming "unusual experiences" (trauma), you may have been predisposed to keep your mouth shut and try to deal with your feelings alone, inside yourself. You may not have chosen to use any opportunities that have presented themselves to ventilate or express your true feelings. You may also have inherited from your family the belief that your feelings of horror, pain, guilt, or anger about the overwhelming things that have happened show that you are a weak or otherwise "not okay" person and therefore have taken steps to hide what you judged as your weakness.

In such a case, the healing path requires not only coming to peace with the overwhelming things that have happened but also coming to peace with those elements of your ancestor inheritance with which you are still at war. This latter part is what I refer to as "healing with ancestors."

Healing with Ancestors: A Story

Robert Ragaini (1986) wrote an essay titled "In My Father's Image," which clearly describes the potentially damaging consequences of the type of hidden inheritance I have been discussing. Although Ragaini discusses only a father/son inheritance, look across the full spectrum of your family of origin for potential inheritances. Ragaini writes:

"Several years ago, I received a terrible shock. Riding on the subway one night, I looked across the aisle and saw my father's face reflected in the darkened window opposite. The face was mine, of course, but it looked to me exactly as my father's had when he was my age. I always knew that I resembled my father, but until then I had been a younger version. Suddenly, I had reached the age that matched the memory I had of him, and when I saw myself in that dusty window, it was he who stared back in disbelief. What was most startling, more even than the uncanny likeness, was the expression. It was his expression, serious, fixed, angry, and it frightened me again as it had when I was a child. It was a sobering experience, to be as old as my father. In his presence I had never felt fully grown up. Now I was looking at the face that had so often intimidated me, and it was my own. The subway car rattled from stop to stop, but I was transfixed by what I had seen. Without knowing it, I had inherited that severe, humorless look, and I didn't want it. Yet there it was. My father was the son of an Italian immigrant tailor — a man I never met and about whom I know almost nothing. I have only one photograph of him. His face is broader than ours, and he's wearing a stiff, round collar and a handlebar mustache and has the familiar furrow between his brows. His name was Atillio, and he died sometime in the 1920's.

"Somehow, my father went from Youngstown, Ohio to Yale University, became a civil engineer, and joined a firm in which he eventually became a partner — where he worked until he retired. He met and married my mother when she was 19, over the objections of her father who didn't approve of Italians.

"Few couples in those days even considered the possibility of a childless marriage, and, in due course, I made my appearance, followed six years later by my brother. And yet, I wonder if my father ever realized how ill-equipped he was for parenthood. What he knew best and valued most was hard work, and almost from the beginning he expected from me more than I could possibly give. So I grew up believing that there was something wrong with me. I was a good boy, obedient, well mannered, and I did well in school, but all that was taken for granted. It was only the failures, the steps backward, that were acknowledged, and I perceived them as monumental sins.

"As I grew older, my father made faltering attempts to come closer. He took me to the theater, attended school functions, but he was unnatural in the role. I believe now that he, too, was frightened, strangely, of me. After all, the standards he set also applied to him and he must have sensed that he wasn't doing very well.

"So far, I've painted a picture of him as a one dimensional, colorless character, but that isn't accurate. I vividly remember parties at our house with friends my parents had known since high school. With them he was easygoing, happy, laughing. At those times he relaxed the rules about bedtime, let me join the party, and treated me as if he actually liked me. These rare breaks in an otherwise unrelieved strictness provided me with my fondest memories of him.

"The subway ride, with its phantom in the window, jarred loose these recollections. I hadn't thought much about my father for some time. When I grew up, my father and I jockeyed for position until we found a kind of fit, but it was never right. The years of my teenage rebellion were behind us, but I was never at ease with him nor he with me. We tried, but we failed. When he died, I grieved and went on. The night before the funeral I was alone with him and said goodbye. The next day I was stunned when several people told me how proud he had been of me. He had never told me.

"I have been absolutely sure of very few things in my life, but one of them was that I did not want to be like my father. But when I saw his look on my face, I had to ask myself just how much of him I was carrying inside me. Had I, like him, become a workaholic? Yes. The boy who bitterly resented the endless chores and jobs was a man who didn't know how to relax. Was I sober, moralistic? Yes. Was I angry? Oh, yes.

"Was there nothing in which I was dissimilar, in which I was my own man? My life was very different from his. I had quit school, determinedly rejected his attitudes, disdained his middle-class lifestyle. Yet, somehow, over the years, the pose had slipped, and I found myself with those very characteristics I had resolved to deny.

"If this was true of me, what about my own son? If I was powerless to avoid my father's influence, had I become a conduit through which it flowed, a direct line between the two? In this context, issues that had confused me seemed clear. My son had been a fearful child. Later, he became sullen, and later still, he often exhibited a kind of anger so familiar to me. I realized that his early fear, which I found alien, was also ours. At that age he simply hadn't had time to convert it fully to anger.

"I believe that there are very few basic feelings in the human repertoire, though the ways we express them are many and varied. The most potent of these is terror, perhaps felt at birth. With love and nurturing, it will not grow out of shape or size, but if reinforced by such things as impossible expectations and parental disapproval, it can dominate and distort its unwilling host. For some, the result is helplessness. These are the frightened, wounded souls we all knew. The men of my family, however, took their terror and forged it into rage and used that rage to hide from the very feeling that drove it.

"Supporting that edifice became a lifelong work, and the effort did awful damage. Enemies were everywhere, and often they were women. Spontaneity was out of the question. Our relationships, especially with each other, were governed by codes that barred any real contact. We knew how to charm, to be likeable, but it was all fraud, and that damned anger ran underneath everything, surfacing unbidden at the slightest provocation.

"I was lucky. Someone who cared enough about me convinced me to seek help. The damage has been done, I can't change my history, but now I have choices I didn't know I had. I know when I'm angry and why I'm angry, and I don't have to let it control me. Sometimes it works.

"For me it was not too late, though much time had been wasted. My son has greater possibilities yet. He carries the family legacy, but he's young, and he has a father who now wants to help. It isn't easy. We have years of tension between us, years of being afraid of each other to overcome.

"For my father, it is too late. He stamped me with his image, and he gave me his pain and then he went away. I wish I missed him more."

As Ragaini's reflections demonstrate, **it is possible to discover elements of our hidden inheritance many years after it has been transmitted.** Such discovery can create more freedom in our lives by opening new choices — choices we may not previously have known were available. Becoming aware of ancestor-inheritance in this way helps in realizing that the method inherited for dealing with anger or other turbulent experiences is only one option out of a wider variety available. With time, and work, he learned to use other options with increased comfort and success.

Choosing to Pay Attention to Unfinished Business

As in all such cases of coming to terms with a hidden inheritance, the first step involved becoming aware, through honest self-appraisal, that something had been inherited. When you are acting a certain way unconsciously, you see, this means that you are not aware that you are acting in that manner or that you could choose to act differently. Therefore, you have little ability to change your style because you simply don't have access to any information that can convincingly demonstrate that how you are acting has something to do with choices that you are making. Once your unconscious actions become conscious, however, and you become aware of the kind of action-strategy you have been using, new possibilities emerge. For the first time you can ask yourself: "Do I act like this because I choose to, or have I been programmed to act like this without knowing I could choose something else instead?"

One place to start in the search for hidden inheritances is by considering the concept of "unfinished business" in your life. "Unfinished business," as I noted in Chapter 8, means just what it sounds like: things left undone, transactions that are somehow incomplete. The best way to know where you have unfinished business in your life experience is by studying your own feelings, as you consider what has happened. Over your lifetime you have had many experiences, and you have likely judged some of them as "good" and others as "bad." This idea of unfinished business with a particular life experience doesn't have much to do with whether you label it a "good" or "bad" experience. Unfinished business means simply that you feel something was left undone.

Let me give an example. Suppose that when you were adolescent you fell in love with someone but were too shy to tell them, and suppose further that no one else has touched your heart in that way since. Whenever you think of this early love you might breathe a wistful sigh of regret for what might have been — there is a strong emotional reaction that draws you off-balance.

Imagine that same situation again, supposing that this time you did express your feelings to your loved one. Perhaps you were flatly rejected; perhaps you had a steaming romance. In either case, you followed your feelings, and a conclusion was reached. When you reminisce about this person now, you can remember your youthful rejection or your youthful romance without feeling that something was left undone. It is not imbalancing to remember this scenario: however it turned out, it feels complete. You do not become ensnared in thinking about might-have-beens when you turn your attention that way. In this situation, there is not unfinished business left behind.

Unfinished business, then, refers to experiences which have happened that you have not yet laid to rest. Perhaps you feel there is something you left unsaid, or undone; perhaps you said or did more than now seems fitting. Whatever the nature of your particular unfinished business, you can question yourself about it once it has been located. Ask yourself, "What did I want to happen, instead of what did happen? What do I regret about how I or someone else acted, then? What don't I regret? What would it take for this to feel completed?"

The answers to these types of questions provide clues that point towards laying unfinished business to rest. You cannot go back and change the past, but you can make choices that incorporate your desires about what happened then into how you live now. In this way, you may gradually come to forgive yourself or others for any mistakes you believe were made. If you tell yourself you are a "bad person" because of how you acted, for example, you may suffer from self-hatred because you don't know how to separate the basic "you" from the actions you took then.

Following this strategy of working on unfinished business, you can learn from the actions you are now judging as "bad." You can learn to admit to yourself that you are a person who judges those actions as "bad," and learn to condemn the actions instead of the person that acted them out in the past. If you do this, you will know that you are now a person who does not choose to act that way. With this knowledge, you can become more able to see yourself as you are now, and forgive yourself for who you were then.

Unfinished business frequently shows up in places where we have received some hidden and unwanted inheritance from our family. It may be useful to go over your exercise notes and see what sort of things that made a difference may have happened in your early life. If you didn't record any events involving your family, then consider them now: is there any unfinished business with your family members? If so, what is the nature of this business? What was left unsaid or undone, or was done to excess? What transpired that you would change now if you could?

The places you locate unfinished business with family members may give you some clues about some of the hidden inheritance you have received from your family. The answers you come up with to the preceding questions may give you some clues about the kinds of things you can do now to lay the unfinished business to rest. In some cases this may involve going back and communicating with those with whom you have left something undone. In other cases, you may need to work the unfinished business out inside yourself.

Not all unfinished business has to do with experiences that are ugly and filled with pain or fear. Sometimes unfinished business can relate to opportunities where you were offered love, beauty, or otherwise spiritually nourishing experiences, but somehow couldn't quite make the connections, or more accurately couldn't bring them to a place where they felt completed. So while in some cases working

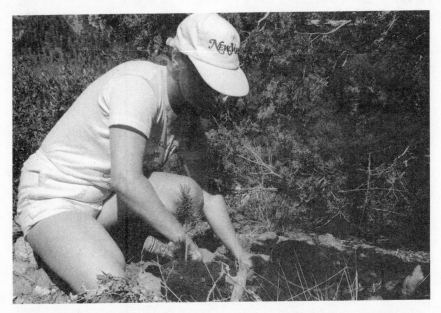

Wilderness volunteer staff planting tree: "unfinished business" at El Descanso Mine,
California Sierras. (photo: Tsolo)

on unfinished business may involve grieving, accepting limitations, and moving away from old ways of doing things, in other cases it may involve opening up to joy and new possibilities and moving towards old ways of doing things.

"Old Ghosts" as Unfinished Business

Healing with ancestors (your inheritance from your family of origin) is really one special case of coming to terms with what has happened in your past. I use the term "old ghosts" to refer to all the things that have happened in the past with which a person has unfinished business.

In myths and legends, "ghosts" are consistently portrayed with several common features: they are difficult to see, they are frightening, and they haunt people. "Old ghosts" from the past — a type of presence lingering on from overwhelming events and other events that made a difference — share these qualities. **Overwhelming things that have happened can influence us as strongly as our family inheritance.**

To locate the places where there is this kind of unfinished business, follow the same line of inquiry that you pursued in looking for unfinished business with your family. When you point your attention that way, there is a strong emotional reaction that draws you off-balance. This is a tip-off or clue that you have not yet come to peace with what has happened. The ways to heal with "old ghosts" are as varied as the experiences such ghosts represent; however, they all involve paying attention to the nature of the unfinished business which is hauntingly present. **Something happened, and in your true heart it still matters.**

If you feel haunted by the memory of a person whose death you experienced, for example, you may need to find a way to sincerely extend peaceful intentions to that dead person in order to obtain a measure of peace yourself. Another way to say this is that these haunting experiences seem to show up in those aspects of our experience where we still really care about something that happened before. This means that our sense of caring — the part of our identity that knows how to love — has somehow been thrown off-balance in relation to what happened then.

Cultivating balance in this situation, what I have been calling "healing with old ghosts," means finding ways to use this loving part of our nature when confronting any "ghosts" that may be haunting our memories. We only feel haunted when we experience an unwanted presence. Where we can find a way to welcome that presence when it shows up in our lives, it ceases to be present in a way that frightens and unbalances us.

One major reason why the Vietnam Veteran's Memorial in Washington, D.C. has been so popular with Vietnam veterans and the American public generally is because it makes available a rare, culturally sanctioned way to come into contact with "old ghosts" from the Vietnam war era. The Wall provides a context where it is okay 1) to mourn what needs to be mourned; 2) to pay attention to the memories of overwhelming events; and 3) to communicate with the presence of those who have died. The Vietnam Veteran's Memorial has become America's most accessible site for initiating the work of "healing with old ghosts."

More recently, a project for incest survivors was carried out in Berkeley, California. It is called the "Healing Wall" and serves a similar function as the Veterans Memorial Wall. In the "Healing Wall" project, one thousand incest survivors were invited to paint one ceramic tile each with a healing image relevant to their experience. In this way a community of grieving and affirmation was likewise convened to provide a place for "healing with old ghosts."

To do this type of work, honesty, patience, and courage are all required. This type of communication can, in time, lead to a "letting go" of the oppressive weight of the burdens that have been carried, enabling new purpose and a reconnection with a sense of caring to emerge for survivors.

I participated in one Vietnam veterans' "rap" group where the veterans were confronted by the question of a group member who had felt plagued by "old ghosts" for many years. This veteran had spent much effort over the past year talking about his war experience for the first time since military service. He had experienced repeated waves of anger, grief, guilt, and sadness about the things that had happened in his life. He was tired of it all, he said, and his question was very simple: "How long? How long do I have to feel like this before it gets better?" Another veteran — a skilled "rap" group facilitator and a man with a good heart (D.C. Hutchinson) who had helped me get groups started in Olympia — gave his reply: "You've got to keep it up until you get tired of it." This simple statement touches on an essential truth about "healing with old ghosts." Since you cannot change what happened before, the only possible place for meaningful change to occur is inside you, the person who is "haunted" in some way by what happened. **You can change your relationship to old events by changing how you are in the world now** — by "getting tired" of maintaining your old pattern of blaming others or yourself for what happened in a way that leaves you feeling "stuck." I do not in any way mean to say that this is easy work; I do want to say loud and clearly that this work is possible, and that there are now many survivors of various qualities of overwhelming experiences who can testify that this is real.

The person who has seemingly unsolvable problems can escape them only when he learns how to no longer be the person with those problems. **Healing involves opening up to new meanings that can be extracted from what happened before, from what is happening now, and from what is possible in the future.** When we find some meaning that we could not find before, this new meaning can shift our sense of who we are to such a degree that we are no longer in the world in the same way as before. Where this occurs, we can say that we have learned how to no longer be the person with those problems, that that person "got tired" of relating in that way and found some meaning that enabled a healing change.

10

Respect and Real Work

All living things have life in common. The more one pays attention to the sameness, the less threatening the differences will appear.

When we give our respect to another human being, we hold them in high regard and consider them important. We pay attention to their point of view. Our respect allows us to see this other person as a valued life. Where we judge a person as deserving of our disrespect, we act quite differently. We do not consider such people important, and we may work very diligently to ignore their point of view. We often do not evaluate the lives of those we disrespect in the same way we evaluate those we respect. The standards we use to decide where we will give our true respect, then, are very important in determining how we will relate to others.

War is an extreme case where whole nations decide to actively disrespect each other's human rights; once this decision has been reached, the other side becomes "the enemy" and for us they are no longer truly human. We do not consider them important, we do not want to understand their point of view, and we do not value their lives. When disrespect runs out of control in this way, wholesale pain and suffering are the inevitable result.

For those who have been exposed to war and other violently overwhelming events, the human tendency towards disrespectful actions may appear as far more real and substantial than the human capacity for respectful action. For example, as one Vietnam veteran stated:

After watching friends die, after seeing body counts get piled up like points in football games, after believing in the rap about "killing Commies for Christ," after coming home and seeing the difference between what was on the airwaves and what was really happening, after being worried about it all and talking to doctors who would only say "stay calm and try to adjust" and offer pills — well, it just got kind of tough to find anything I could respect.

Similarly, as one rape survivor stated:

After I got raped I was very frightened, and later angry, to know that this could happen to me, anytime, anywhere. I went all over the system looking for some support, some protection, something to help me deal with the sense of violation. I couldn't believe how many places I encountered the attitude that: "If you didn't protect yourself better than that, you must have wanted it." It felt like the Dark Ages, and I lost all respect for our society's ability to care for women.

Cultivating Balance by Practicing Respect

Respect occurs when we hold a person, an ideal, or anything else in high regard: when the object of our respect is somehow favorably connected to something that matters, something we really care about. **It can become increasingly difficult to maintain contact with one's sense of respect in environments where disrespect appears as the rule rather than the exception.**

Disrespect is among our most powerful psychological tools in dehumanizing anyone whose needs we choose to ignore. With sufficient use and insufficient exposure to alternatives, like any mental habit it can become an addiction.

When we respectfully hold someone or something in high regard, we send signals that we value their aliveness and that we are glad that they exist. The other person, thing, or nation, watching how we treat them, gradually comes to know of our respectful intentions. When we show disrespect, however, we send signals that the other person or nation is not okay, that we feel we are justified in our desire to change or condemn them. As they watch our actions, they come to fear our intolerant judgments, since such judgments question their freedom to be as they are.

The fear created by disrespectful actions leads to disrespectful reactions, which creates more fear. This is the all-too-well-known spiral that leads to confrontations and war — in relationships, in families, in organizations, and between nations. Respect generates a favorable climate for peace; disrespect generates a favorable climate for war.

In our personal lives, our ability to hold various living things in high regard (other individuals, other races, our planet, and ourselves) is intimately connected with our ability to experience peace. If you love nature and hate the human race, for example, it's a safe bet that you won't go to the local social club when you need to be emotionally refreshed. You'll go somewhere in nature, because you hold her in high regard and therefore can feel safe relaxing and letting your guard down in that presence. The less that we find in our lives that we can hold in high regard, the more difficult it's going to be to find places to "let go" of our protective stance and feel at peace. Our inner war, then, and our inner peace, are in large part determined by the positions we have taken concerning respect. Where it is "tough to find anything to respect," it is likely also very difficult to experience peace.

All living things have life in common. This means we are all connected by the same experience. The more one pays attention to the sameness, the less threatening appear the differences. The vast majority of all spiritual traditions in all cultures throughout history emphasize the quality of universal respect as a high achievement in cultivating balance. It is also emphasized in the motto appearing as the standard of the United States on every coin in the realm: "E pluribus unum," which when translated from Latin to English means "from many, one."

If the idea of universal respect is too large a mouthful for you to chew on all at once, you can still stake out a little beachhead on the island of your choice to which you can give your respect. As you give yourself permission to apply your own high regard, it can teach you useful ways to experience peace. Little by little, you may acquire further real estate where you can invest your respect to good effect. Your dividends are greater freedom to experience peace inside and outside yourself, depending on the quality of the investments you make.

Disrespect and Ability to Experience Peace

The term "nonpeace" has been used by some to distinguish between those actions that lead towards peaceful processes and those which do not. For individuals the simple declaration of being "for peace" is insufficient to guard against nonpeaceful actions because so many of our actions are based on unconscious beliefs that are outside our awareness. To guard against war it is necessary to examine the actions we take and search out those that contribute to nonpeace. **As we learn to pay attention to our nonpeaceful actions, other options become available.**

The situations where we contribute to nonpeace are those in which we do not extend our respect. If, for example, we hate men or women, or blacks or whites, we will not hold the members of that group in high regard. We will not be able to see them accurately as individuals; our disrespect will help us to ignore their point of view. Disrespect is usually perceived as threatening by those who receive it. Once threatened, their "fight or flight" reactions may be activated, mobilizing them for war. This type of movement closer to an imbalanced use of force is why we can say that our disrespect contributes to nonpeace.

For those highly sensitized by exposure to war or other experiences where human disrespect has been very dominant, it may require contact with that which is most profoundly peaceful and sacred in human experience to provide the focus necessary in rekindling the flame of high regard. One traumatized veteran of a foreign war, coming home from the combat zone and finding difficulty in respecting the established order of the day, found a measure of peace by cultivating deep respect for all living things. His war was the Crusades, and he became known as St. Francis of Assisi. Other cases abound throughout human history, connecting cultures, continents, and centuries. Various writers have discussed the experience of "warrior ship" in referring to the shift that can occur when nonpeaceful experiences are used as a learning ground to motivate the acquisition of deep respect.

If in working towards peace it is useful to ask what we do that contributes to nonpeace, then in working towards respect it may be necessary to question ourselves about the things we do that are disrespectful — to those we see as enemies, to ourselves, to our families, our nation, and our planet. This type of rigorous questioning can illuminate the darkest corners of our hearts and minds and help change occur naturally. And the answers to this type of inquiry do not come only from the questions posed by our intellectual mind — they also emerge from the silence of our meditations and the metaphors given in our daily life.

Spiritual Growth as "Real Work"

Cultivating deep balance in these ways has formed the basis of the work of spiritual traditions around the world. Though methods and myths have varied dramatically, there is nearly universal agreement among those who have taught about the refinement of human consciousness that the ability to cultivate respect is a potential for all human beings. I like to refer to this type of activity as "real work."

"Real work" may or may not have anything to do with any jobs you may perform to earn what you need to survive. Working at any particular type of employment may or may not be "real work," depending on whether or not you can respect the task you are engaged in. "Real work" may or may not involve material compensation or recognition from the outside. **Real work" is any activity you choose to become involved with because it helps you feel more alive and connected to your sense of purpose.** We locate our "real work" in those domains where we have the highest regard; that is, where we give our deepest respect.

It is very important to remember that the consequences of overwhelming events can include a spiritual crisis. That is, one's previous concept of deity, or the sacred, or the spiritual dimension as otherwise conceived, can be deeply affected. The story or personal myth that an individual has been telling themselves about their relationship to the sacred may somehow be called into question by what happened. Where was God when this happened? How can I believe in some intangible principle of connectedness when I have experienced such profoundly divisive disrespect, where the lack of connectedness was so apparent?

No external source holds a monopoly on the most valid answers to an individual's questions about their relationship to the spiritual dimension. I am saying that it is important to acknowledge that this is one of the domains where our "life tree" may have needed to stretch in some unusual directions in order to adapt to our personal situation. **The question of the apparently absent God and the inability to experience connection with the sacred are themes of**

spiritual crisis. Following these themes can bring us to awareness of our unhealed wounds in the spirit, to those places where we have experienced deep loss, to the places where we can now find meaningful connection in pursuing our own "real work." There is a theme that exists across the spiritual psychologies of many cultures that the healing journey leads through the "dark night of the soul," through the places where these losses live, in order to reforge our spiritual connections. This is the essence of renewal, to literally make new again the life of our spirit.

Interestingly, in this year 1992 for the first time a diagnostic category has been proposed to the American Psychological Association of "psychospiritual disorder." Although it may be many years yet before this type of thinking about human nature becomes widely accepted in our health delivery systems, it is nonetheless an early indication of a growing acknowledgement that this realm of our human experience is important, is relevant to our health, and should not be ignored.

It is my sincere hope that by this point in your explorations you have recalled some aspect or aspects of your experience that you can hold in high regard. These are good starting points in your search for "real work" that is relevant to you. Trusting your own power to sense when something matters to you can enable you to connect to activities that are meaningful. "Real work" is about the type of mission you can choose with an open heart to connect you through your actions to the motion of life.

Building Healing Community

Throughout this book I have been discussing mostly the steps along a healing journey that can be taken in isolation, on a solitary walk. I felt the need to speak this way because I have seen that the "life trees" of many survivors have stretched their roots and branches in ways that require considerable isolation.

It should be said that when it comes to this subject of respect and "real work," the isolated walk is not the whole story. There are things you can do because you are your own individual "life tree," and there are other things you can do because you are part of a forest, an ecosystem, a community. **Finding the places in your life where you can build healing community is very nourishing, and this quality of nourishment can play a major role in giving you the strength**

you need to take the difficult steps along the solitary parts of your journey. I have alluded to just a few possibilities concerning how the healing journeys of individuals can come together to form community: in therapy groups, in peer survivor sharing, in dreamwork groups, in meditation and martial arts training, in healing with ancestors and old ghosts, in creative ceremonies offering prayers for peaceful rest, in using your voice to offer compassion to others, in choosing to acknowledge connection with the earth. All of these actions are choices about where to invest your respect. The places you can find to willingly invest your high regard in support of others are your "natural ecosystem" and hold clues about the places you are most likely to be able to form healing community.

Healing Use of the Self in Society

There is one last point I would like to make in discussing the relations between trauma, peace, and post-traumatic experience. As I stated in Chapter 2, a healing strategy that promotes "readjustment" is insufficient to address in a meaningful way the questions raised by exposure to massive disrespect. Such a strategy sees people who have lost their balance after such exposure as diseased victims of a medical disorder. There is an additional quality often observable in trauma survivors, which is rarely noted in the medical literature. Such literature often catalogues observations of anger episodes, anxiety, vigilance, and paranoid thinking and views people who have been exposed to massive disrespect in terms of their deficiencies and inability to act "normally."

When we think in terms of the previous discussion about peace and nonpeace, respect and disrespect, however, we can develop a different point of view. Individuals who have been exposed to profound disrespect are extrasensitive when they find themselves in environments where disrespectful actions are occurring. They react to even the most subtle forms of nonpeace more rapidly and with greater energy than the general population.

Although it is true we can look at this difference from a point of view that judges it as disease, it is equally possible to view this difference from another point of view. Post-traumatic stress reactions are frequently triggered by the presence of nonpeace (disrespectful actions) in the environment of traumatized individuals. This means that the reactions seen in post-traumatic distress are in part measurements of the peaceful vs. nonpeaceful content of the actions in the environment. Another way to say this is that such individuals possess heightened sensitivity concerning when nonpeaceful intentions and actions are present.

To be extrasensitive to the presence of nonpeace is to have increased ability to pay attention effectively when disrespectful actions are occurring. It is a tragic comment on the state of the times that for so many suffering from post-traumatic distress, environments that are deeply peaceful have not been located. As more and more of those who have been overwhelmed by the disrespect in our human world find their way along a healing path, their voices may increasingly be heard speaking in favor of respectful actions leading towards peace.

Survivors of profound disrespect have much to teach about the hidden and subtle forms of nonpeace that are so difficult for all of us to recognize in ourselves. Those who find "real work" in service of promoting peace and reducing fear inside themselves and in the world will truly find their lives again infused with purpose and an opening heart.

About the Author

Benjamin Colodzin, Ph.D., humanistic psychologist and educator, is founder and director of Olympia Institute. He has worked extensively with Vietnam veterans and veterans of the Afghanistan war.

Olympia Institute is a nonprofit educational organization teaching self-help methods to those affected by exposure to psychologically overwhelming events. Using a multicultural approach, Olympia Institute seeks to design and teach traumatic stress recovery curricula that can be easily assimilated and replicated by the groups that will use them. For information about the programs and activities of Olympia Institute and their availability in your area, contact :

Dr. Benjamin Colodzin
Olympia Institute
P.O. Box 750
Bolinas, California 94924

Good Grief Rituals
Tools for Healing
ELAINE CHILDS-GOWELL

As a psychotherapist with over 20 year's experience, the author realized that the emotion of grief was not limited to bereavement but was in fact experienced in an extraordinary range of circumstances, from natural disasters to the end of a love affair. In this sane, comforting, and deeply thoughtful book, she offers the reader a series of simple grief rituals, among them the venting of feelings, letter writing, affirmations, exercises to act out negative emotions as well as forgiveness, fantasies, meditations, and more. Adult children of alcoholics and dysfunctional families, victims of incest and assault, and those who've lost a beloved or a pet, wrecked a car, or suffered any kind of loss, will find that these "good grief rituals" move them through loss to forgiveness and, ultimately, to gratitude and a new sense of life.

$8.95 paper, ISBN 0-88268-118-4

Emotional First Aid
A Crisis Handbook
SEAN HALDANE, M.D.

Emotional First Aid is the first book to address immediate emotional crisis as distinct from a person's general state of mental health. It deals with grief, anger, fear, joy, and also the complex feelings of parent/child conflicts—emotions that can lead to further withdrawal, illness, or even violence. Clear and extraordinarily well written, this is the first book to draw on Reichian character analysis to explain how differences in individuals and in specific emotions call for different responses, if one is to be supportive and not invasive. Emotional first aid may precede or prevent therapy in the same way that physical first aid can precede or prevent extended medical treatment.

$9.95 paper, ISBN 0-88268-071-4

How to Forgive
When You Don't Know How
JACQUI BISHOP AND MARY GRUNTE

In this groundbreaking look at the psychology of forgiveness, the authors show how resentment toward other people, toward one's self, even toward God can consume precious emotional energy and seriously impair both self-esteem and the ability to experience joy. Drawing on the healing techniques used so successfully in *How to Love Yourself When You Don't Know How*, they offer a short program for accelerating the process of forgiveness, including visualization, emotional discharge, searching back, and prayer. Envlivened with classic quotations on the nature of forgiveness, this revolutionary book explodes long-standing myths including the notion that forgiveness involves self-denial, making up, confessing, or turning the other cheek. Its easy-to-use format puts it on the shelf with *Good Grief Rituals*.

$8.95 paper, ISBN 0-88268-142-7

How to Love Yourself
When You Don't Know How
Healing All Your Inner Children
JACQUI BISHOP AND MARY GRUNTE

The notion that each of us carries around an inner child has been widely explored in popular psychology; this groundbreaking book takes the premise one step further, describing an interior model for the individual based on the metaphor of the family. Everyone, say the authors, is really made up of an inner family—several children of various ages and characters, each of whom vies for control in one's life, as well as an inner grown-up capable of learning to care for them. The book's aim is to help the reader re-educate the inner grownup to love unconditionally, opening the way for profound healing of psychic wounds.

$10.95 paper, ISBN 0-88268131-1

How To Break the Vicious Circles in Your Relationships

A Guide for Couples

DEE ANNA PARRISH, MSSW

The message of this clear and sympathetic book is that dysfunctional relationships—characterized by a predictable pattern of vicious circles—can be healed. Reassuring case histories drawn from the author's own therapeutic practice demonstrate why relationships disintegrate and show how they can be made whole again. Here are proven techniques designed to short-circuit destructive habits. Readers will learn to use "defusers" to keep conflicts from escalating, gauge levels of emotional intimacy and identify barriers to closeness, examine their own levels of communication and quality of listening, use "I" statements to identify problematic issues, and uncover inter-generational patterns of dysfunction. For anyone seeking to improve a relationship or reconnect with a partner—with or without the aid of a therapist—this is essential reading.

$8.95 paper, ISBN 0-88268-144-3

Abused

A Guide to Recovery for Adult Survivors of Emotional/Physical Child Abuse

DEE ANNA PARRISH, MSSW

This clear and sensitively written book covers child abuse in all its forms, including types of abuse overlooked by the victims themselves: neglect, deprivation, ridicule, and inappropriate sexual gestures. *Abused* includes a wealth of revealing and highly moving first-person accounts, a program for recovery, a resource directory, and various self-tests to help readers determine if they once were abused and today need counselling or therapy. It includes a parents' guide to behavioral signs of sexual abuse plus the first guide to describe techniques used by therapists to uncover repressed memories. Illustrated with case histories, *Abused* is written for adults who suspect the treatment they received as children still impairs their sense of judgment and well-being today.

$8.95 paper, ISBN 0-88268-089-7

These titles are available from your local bookstore or directly from:
Station Hill Press
Barrytown, New York 12507
Write for a free catalogue